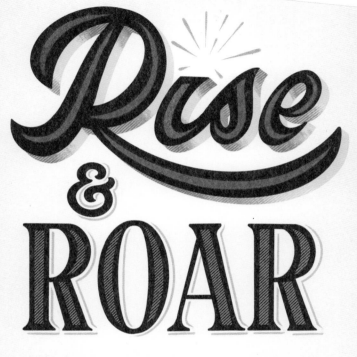

Rise & ROAR

A GUIDED JOURNAL FOR OUTDOOR ADVENTURE

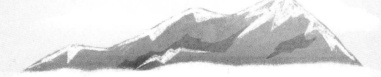

SHARISSE STEBER

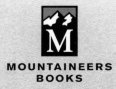

MOUNTAINEERS
BOOKS

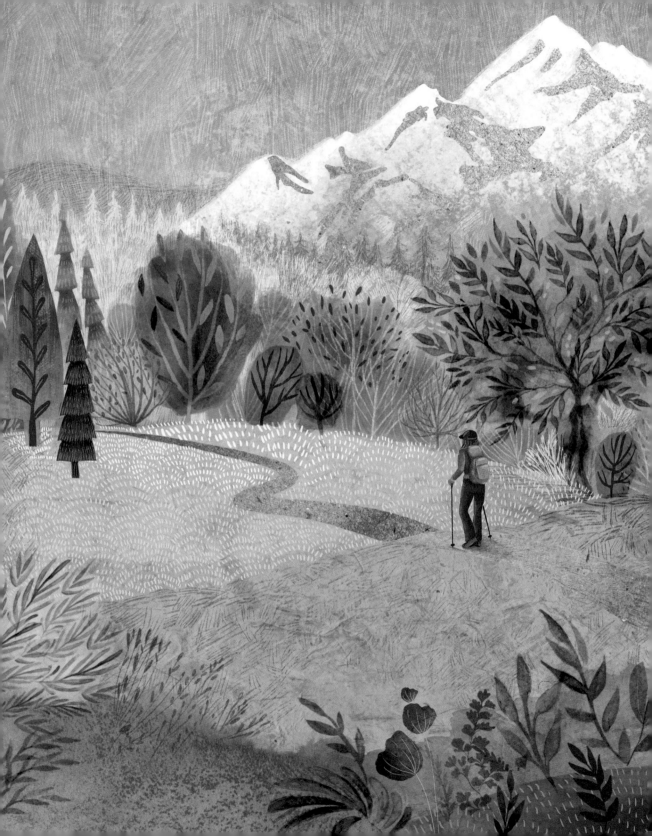

MAKE ROOM FOR MORE OUTDOOR ADVENTURE IN YOUR LIFE!

Are you already a free-spirited, outdoorsy adventure-seeker, or are you a more timid newbie, curious to experience what you see on Instagram? No matter your starting point, there are so many ways to introduce more fun and excitement into your life. You don't have to quit your job and travel the world (although that might be your ultimate dream). Begin where you are now. The days are long, but the years are short. **You still have time to lead the outdoor life you've always wanted.**

I enjoy working as a professional illustrator and graphic designer. My deepest loves, however, are sketching while perched on a rock overlooking a lush valley, reaching a high summit, squeezing through a cave, and whitewater rafting down a river. I always make time for the outdoors, and I want to encourage other women to overcome any fears and explore their inner wild child. From backpacking solo through foreign countries to going on wilderness adventures with my son, I know firsthand that **you don't have to be super fit, wealthy, or free of obligations to live boldly outside.**

Incorporate adventure into your life in a way that works for you. You may long for outdoor freedom but have family responsibilities to consider. Remember, your kids will be young only a short while; make lasting memories canoeing or hiking with them, even as you plan and prepare for your dream trip. My most adventurous life experiences have happened after the age of forty. **The key is to connect to what matters to you now.**

Use this journal to inspire yourself to try new things and plan to make them a reality. You may want to hike more or wish your family would camp more often, or perhaps you dream of climbing a peak or trying downhill skiing for the first time. What matters is that you envision the life you want—and take steps to make that life your own.

Don't be afraid to start small, step outside, breathe deeply, and feel the sun on your face. Then, when you're ready, **GO SEEK ADVENTURE!**

See you on the trail,

Sharisse Steber

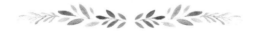

WE ALL HAVE TWO LIVES.
THE SECOND ONE STARTS
WHEN WE REALIZE
WE HAVE ONLY ONE.

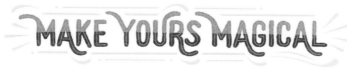

MAKE YOURS MAGICAL

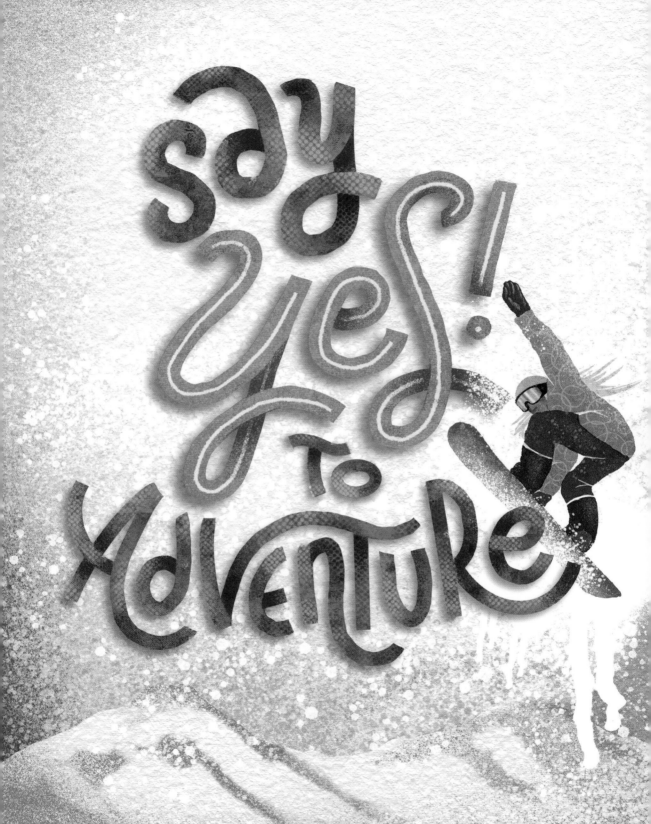

ADVENTURE PLEDGE

Today is the
day I will
BEGIN.

I am curious about the world and want
more adventure in my life.

I will experience nature in new ways and be
open to the **THRILL** of the outdoors.
I don't know everything about how to start,
but I will allow more wind in my hair and sun
on my face as I jump into brave

NEW EXPERIENCES.

I will live with **NO REGRETS** starting **NOW.**

YOUR NAME AND DATE

SHARE YOUR BEAUTY AND RAISE YOUR VOICE

This journal is a place to keep track of your outdoor and adventure dreams. Alongside inspirational profiles of amazing women, I share outdoor tips and ideas based on my experiences. These prompts are meant strictly as jumping-off points, encouraging you to set intentions for your own version of an adventurous life.

I've organized the journal by a number of larger topics and activities. You can explore these in order, dip in and out, or focus on the area that interests you the most. However you decide to use this journal, begin with the initial sections about goals, types of adventure, fears and doubts, and body image. Doing this groundwork now will make your explorations more meaningful.

How do you define an adventurous life?

Have you ever accomplished something adventurous that you were really proud of?

Why do you want to live more adventurously? What fears are holding you back?

Jot down some ideas of how you think the outdoors might change or improve your life. Are your priorities exercise and health? Mental stimulation? A path toward mindfulness? Deeper relationships? Confidence? Pure fun? Or something else?

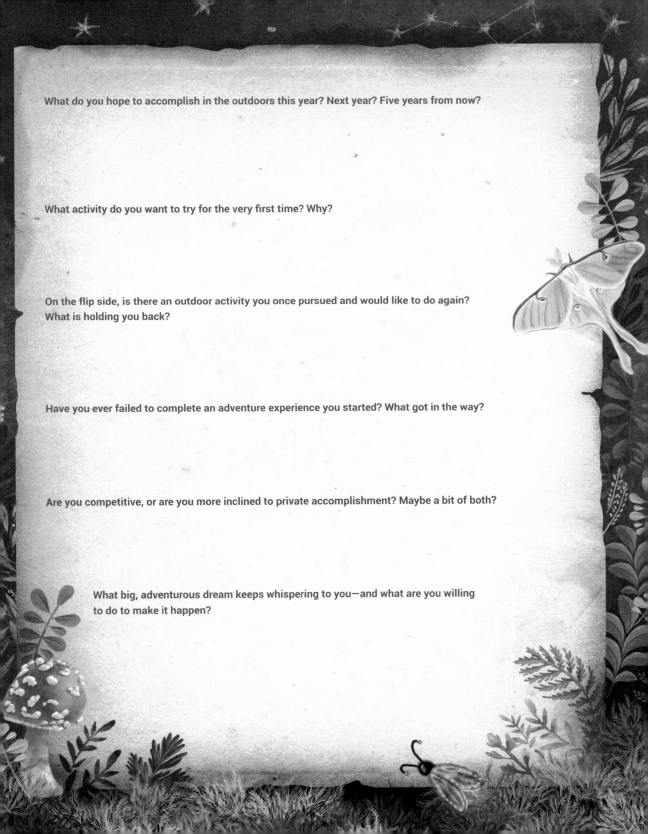

What do you hope to accomplish in the outdoors this year? Next year? Five years from now?

What activity do you want to try for the very first time? Why?

On the flip side, is there an outdoor activity you once pursued and would like to do again? What is holding you back?

Have you ever failed to complete an adventure experience you started? What got in the way?

Are you competitive, or are you more inclined to private accomplishment? Maybe a bit of both?

What big, adventurous dream keeps whispering to you—and what are you willing to do to make it happen?

WHAT KIND OF ADVENTURER ARE YOU?

Do you share any of these traits?

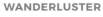

WANDERLUSTER

Every tab in her browser is a search for the latest travel deals. She books a treehouse hotel in the rainforest while on her Arctic expedition in Svalbard. This traveler has a nearly full passport and the wildest tales to share at the hostel. Circling the globe is not a dream, it's her PLAN.

NERVOUS NEWBIE

Becoming out-doorsy is her goal, though she's a bit overwhelmed by how to begin. Determined to leave her comfort zone, she trades a gym session for a hike in the local park. She's over-packed and anxious but thrilled about her first camping trip with friends. She knows the reward is bigger than her fear of the unknown and any rookie mistakes she may make along the way.

LIST-LOVER

The only thing more exhilarating than keeping a running list of places to visit and activities to do is checking them off as accomplished! This type A personality has all her gear neatly organized and categorized. Her planner is filled with goals, dreams, and notes for how to improve. She's an ACTION taker, NOT an excuse maker!

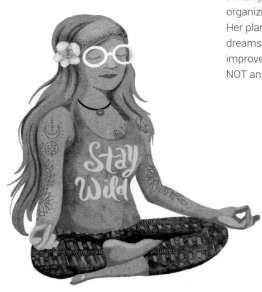

FREE SPIRIT

This magic moonchild runs off to Bali for a yoga retreat and will climb a volcano at sunrise just to do a Sun Salutation in the clouds. She is an adventure goddess who swims under waterfalls then sips an avocado smoothie. Her motto: Good vibes only!

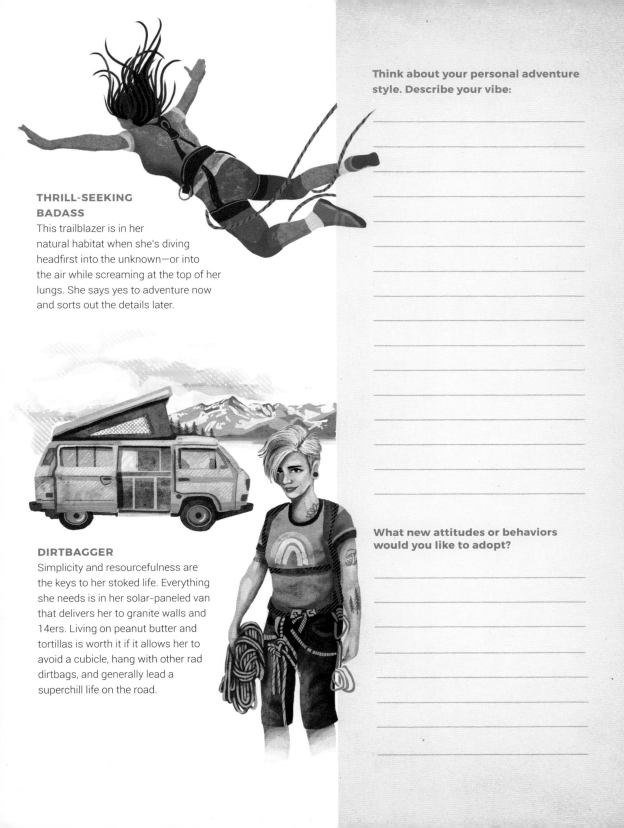

THRILL-SEEKING BADASS

This trailblazer is in her natural habitat when she's diving headfirst into the unknown—or into the air while screaming at the top of her lungs. She says yes to adventure now and sorts out the details later.

DIRTBAGGER

Simplicity and resourcefulness are the keys to her stoked life. Everything she needs is in her solar-paneled van that delivers her to granite walls and 14ers. Living on peanut butter and tortillas is worth it if it allows her to avoid a cubicle, hang with other rad dirtbags, and generally lead a superchill life on the road.

Think about your personal adventure style. Describe your vibe:

_____
_____
_____
_____
_____
_____
_____
_____
_____
_____
_____
_____
_____
_____
_____
_____
_____
_____

What new attitudes or behaviors would you like to adopt?

_____
_____
_____
_____
_____
_____
_____
_____
_____
_____

BUCKET LIST BREAKDOWN

The most effective way to reach any goal is to break it down into bite-sized, achievable chunks. Not only can this reduce anxiety over how to begin, it will help you map out a realistic plan for training and preparation. Here is a sample breakdown of the bucket list goal "Complete Long-Distance Hike." (See the backpacking section for more about the Ten Essentials and other tips.)

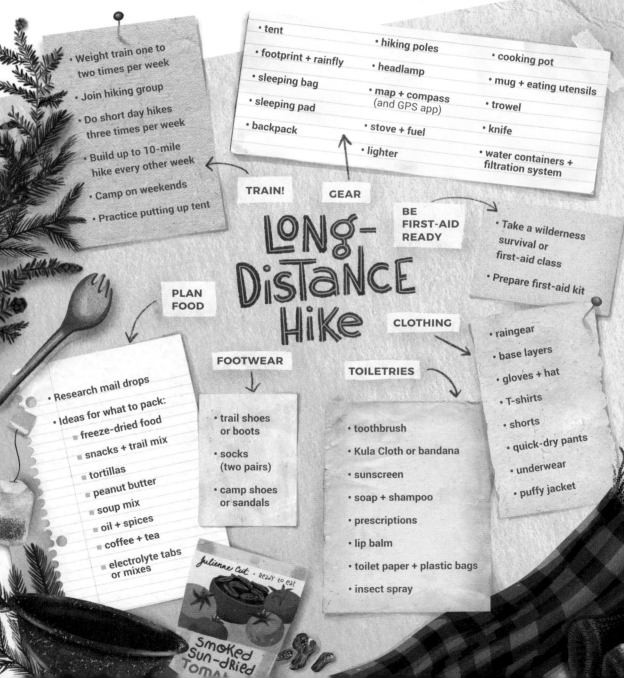

TRAIN!
- Weight train one to two times per week
- Join hiking group
- Do short day hikes three times per week
- Build up to 10-mile hike every other week
- Camp on weekends
- Practice putting up tent

GEAR
- tent
- footprint + rainfly
- sleeping bag
- sleeping pad
- backpack
- hiking poles
- headlamp
- map + compass (and GPS app)
- stove + fuel
- lighter
- cooking pot
- mug + eating utensils
- trowel
- knife
- water containers + filtration system

BE FIRST-AID READY
- Take a wilderness survival or first-aid class
- Prepare first-aid kit

LONG-DISTANCE HIKE

PLAN FOOD
- Research mail drops
- Ideas for what to pack:
  - freeze-dried food
  - snacks + trail mix
  - tortillas
  - peanut butter
  - soup mix
  - oil + spices
  - coffee + tea
  - electrolyte tabs or mixes

FOOTWEAR
- trail shoes or boots
- socks (two pairs)
- camp shoes or sandals

TOILETRIES
- toothbrush
- Kula Cloth or bandana
- sunscreen
- soap + shampoo
- prescriptions
- lip balm
- toilet paper + plastic bags
- insect spray

CLOTHING
- raingear
- base layers
- gloves + hat
- T-shirts
- shorts
- quick-dry pants
- underwear
- puffy jacket

Julienne Cut · Ready to eat

SMOKED SUN-DRIED TOMAT

GETTING STARTED

Beginner basics blogs, guidebooks, and how-to videos are great places to research your activity or destination. Personally, I get inspired following YouTube adventure vloggers who have already accomplished my goal. Watching them pack or organize food drops for a thru-hike, climb a mountain on my bucket list, or describe a trekking itinerary helps me visualize and plan my journey as well as learn from their mistakes.

Pick your own bucket list goal and lay out the steps for your success.

See if your local outfitter offers introductory classes about backpacking, wilderness first aid, navigation, or backcountry cooking. Local meetup groups for hiking, biking, camping, caving, skiing, and kayaking will connect you with mentors willing to share their knowledge. Climbing gyms often organize guided trips to nearby crags. Check out organizations such as Outdoor Women's Alliance and Flash Foxy, and sign up for local events with other women who share your outdoor interests. Don't be intimidated by what you don't know. There are a lot of resources to help you get outdoors!

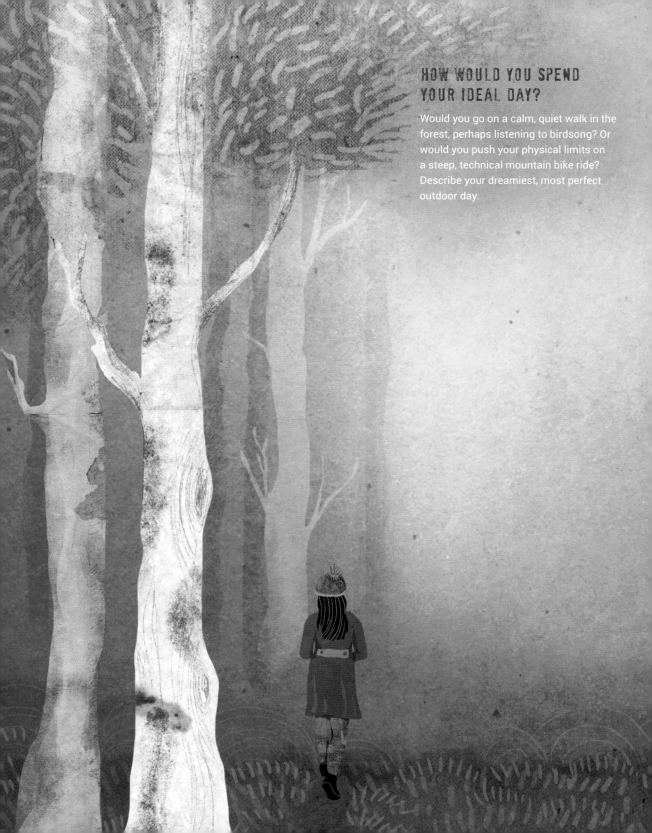

HOW WOULD YOU SPEND YOUR IDEAL DAY?

Would you go on a calm, quiet walk in the forest, perhaps listening to birdsong? Or would you push your physical limits on a steep, technical mountain bike ride? Describe your dreamiest, most perfect outdoor day.

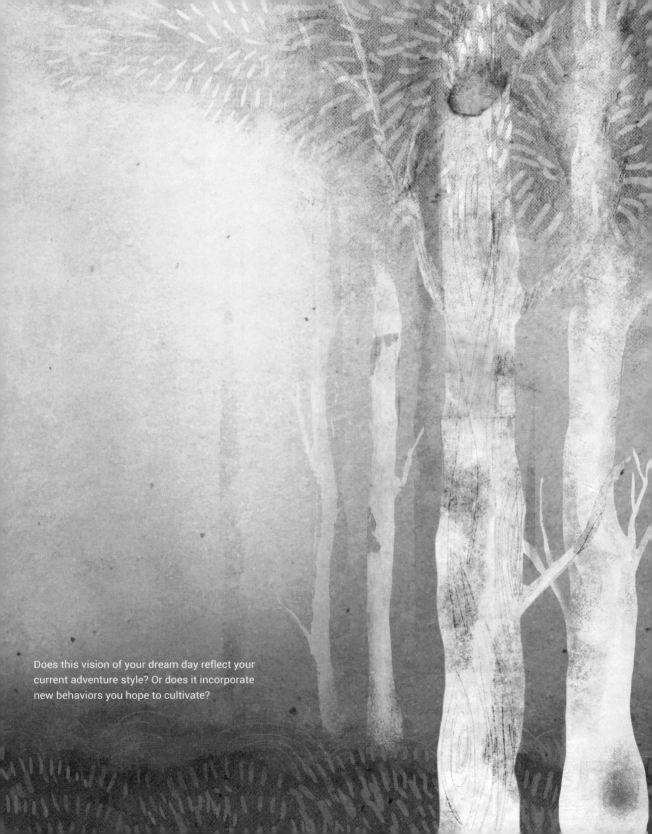

Does this vision of your dream day reflect your current adventure style? Or does it incorporate new behaviors you hope to cultivate?

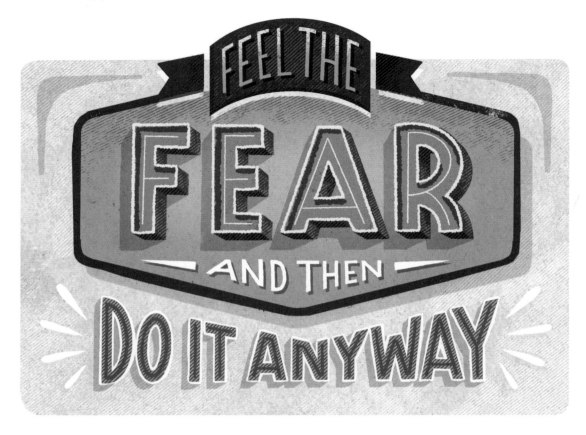

FEEL THE FEAR AND THEN —AND THEN— DO IT ANYWAY

Fear and self-doubt are common, especially in outdoor recreation. Sometimes these concerns come from your loved ones: you've been dreaming about hiking that 200-mile trail or traveling abroad solo, but your friends or family beg you not to go alone. More often the fear comes from within—and can be justified. Even if you're close to home or in an established park, wilderness is still WILDERNESS! There may be thorny plants, poisonous snakes, dangerous animals, slippery footing, or other people who might make you feel unsafe. Have similar worries kept you from your dreams?

The best way to unpack fear is to name it. Once you identify what is holding you back, you can plan effective ways to overcome or minimize each concern so you can live more bravely.

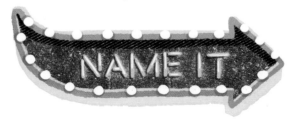

NAME IT

What are your biggest fears about being in the outdoors? Do well-meaning family members or friends sow self-doubt? Do your fears revolve around things under your control, such as your skill level, or things out of your control like wildlife encounters and weather conditions?

How realistic are your fears?
Are these perceived dangers detailed in a guidebook?
Do you have the necessary skills for what you're
hoping to accomplish?

**How would you feel if you never pursued
your outdoor ambition or visited your dream
destination?** Visualize accomplishing that goal
and describe how it makes you feel.

What can you do to address each concern?
For instance, if you are worried about getting injured
in the backcountry, you can carry a satellite communicator, such as a Garmin inReach, that allows you to
send updates to your loved ones and call for help in
an emergency.

One of the biggest challenges of being adventurous
is when well-meaning people who care for you try
to discourage your plans because of their own fears
and limitations. Be ready to stand resolute with a
strong conviction to pursue your dreams.
**Write down what motivates you and repeat
it like a mantra.**

REFRAME YOUR FEARS

Turn each one into a positive intention. A few examples:

"I'm afraid to go alone" becomes "I get a chance
  to focus on me."

"What if I get lost?" becomes "I have a GPS
  app on my phone and the trails are marked."

"Is it safe?" becomes "I can research and prepare."

"What if I get hurt?" becomes "I left my itinerary
  with a friend who knows when to expect me home."

"What if things don't go as planned?" becomes "Seren-
  dipity often leads to more meaningful experiences!"

**List three of your fears and reframe them
in a more positive way.**

FEEL GRATITUDE FOR YOUR BODY

Learn how to love your TODAY body! Starting with your head, think about each body part all the way down to your feet. For each one, briefly note how you feel it is weak and how you *know* it is strong—how each part contributes to your effort to hike, bike, paddle, ski, climb, or pursue any other activity.

BODY PART	WEAKNESS	STRENGTH
Head, eyes, ears		
Neck		
Shoulders		
Upper arms		
Forearms		
Wrists, hands, fingers		
Chest		
Core		
Back		
Glutes and hamstrings		
Knees		
Calves		
Ankles		
Feet and toes		

JENNIFER PHARR DAVIS

RECORD-SETTING HIKER AND BACKPACKER

Jennifer Pharr Davis has hiked more than 14,000 miles on six continents. In 2011 she completed the Appalachian Trail in 46 days, 11 hours, and 20 minutes, setting a Fastest Known Time (FKT). Davis is a hiker, backpacker, and National Geographic Adventurer of the Year who knows that spending time outdoors can be transformative. Despite her record-breaking accomplishments, she recognizes that focusing on numbers and results can be negative and emotionally toxic.

"The thing I miss the most after my first thru-hike—I missed how beautiful I felt out here. When I started, I had accepted all the ways my body was wrong and that I had to forgive. And then I went hiking and it totally changed. All of a sudden being super flat—I'm ultralight. Now I LOVE my body. It wasn't wrong. I didn't have to make apologies for what wasn't standard. You don't have a mirror. I always thought that nature was beautiful, but I had never considered myself part of nature and of all this beauty. So I'm not going to look at the magazines. I'm going to look around and feel connected to this forest and I'm going to feel beautiful."

TAKE A SELFIE AND PLACE IT HERE TO REMIND YOURSELF OF THE GRATITUDE YOU FEEL FOR YOUR BODY AND ALL THAT IT IS CAPABLE OF.

Write a love note to your body.
Describe all the things you're grateful for, all the adventures your body makes possible, and all the ways you hope to stay strong and healthy. Most women struggle with body issues. Do you look at your thighs and see them as too jiggly? Instead, think of how they power you up a steep mountain or cycle a gorgeous trail. Does gratitude change how you see your perceived flaws?

SCRAPBOOK YOUR FUTURE

Reflect on your outdoor goals and create a scrapbook page to represent the future, ten or even twenty years from now. What adventures do you hope to have accomplished? How old will you be? Where will you be?

Using photos, illustrations, drawings, and notes from magazines or websites, create a visual representation of your future experiences. Get creative. Add fun details such as a pressed flower or a leaf from a trail you hope to hike, or glue on sand to represent a desert camping trip you'll take with friends. Visualization is key to making your dreams a reality.

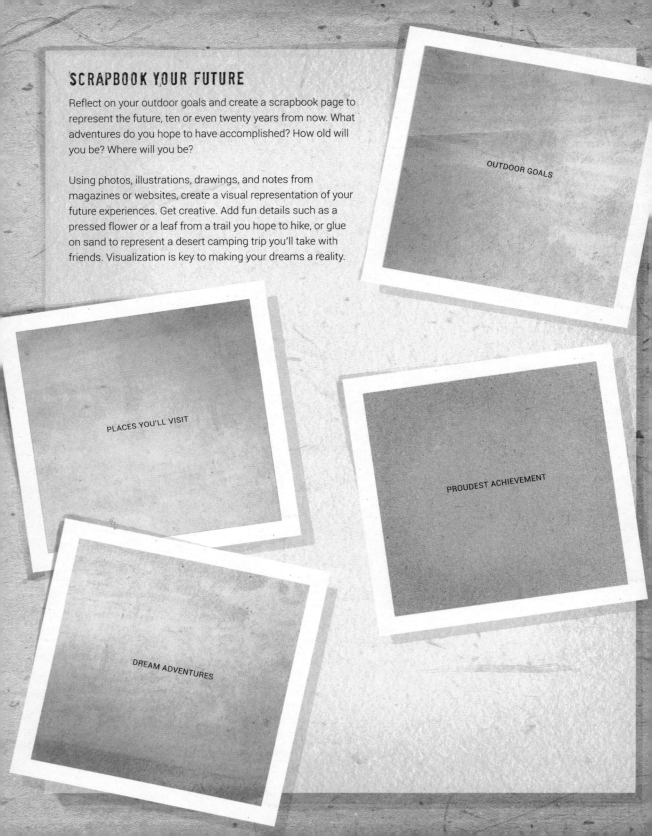

OUTDOOR GOALS

PLACES YOU'LL VISIT

PROUDEST ACHIEVEMENT

DREAM ADVENTURES

CREATE YOUR ADVENTURE MANIFESTO

A manifesto is a declaration of intention for how you want to live. Using brief, declarative sentences or phrases, write (or draw) your own outdoor manifesto. Here's some inspiration to get you started!

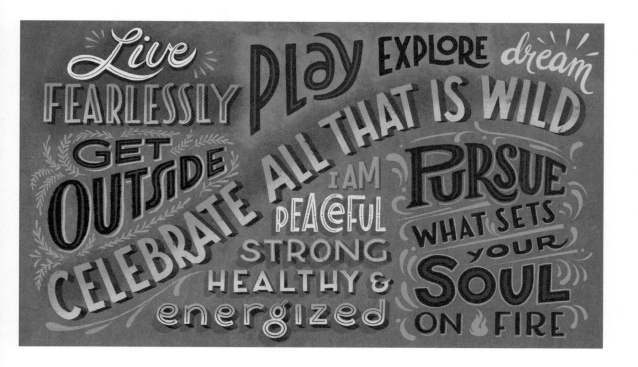

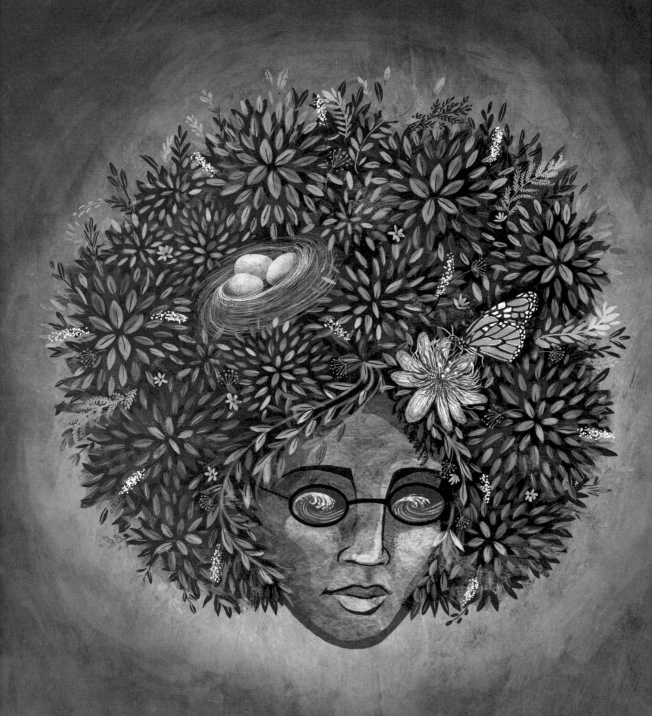

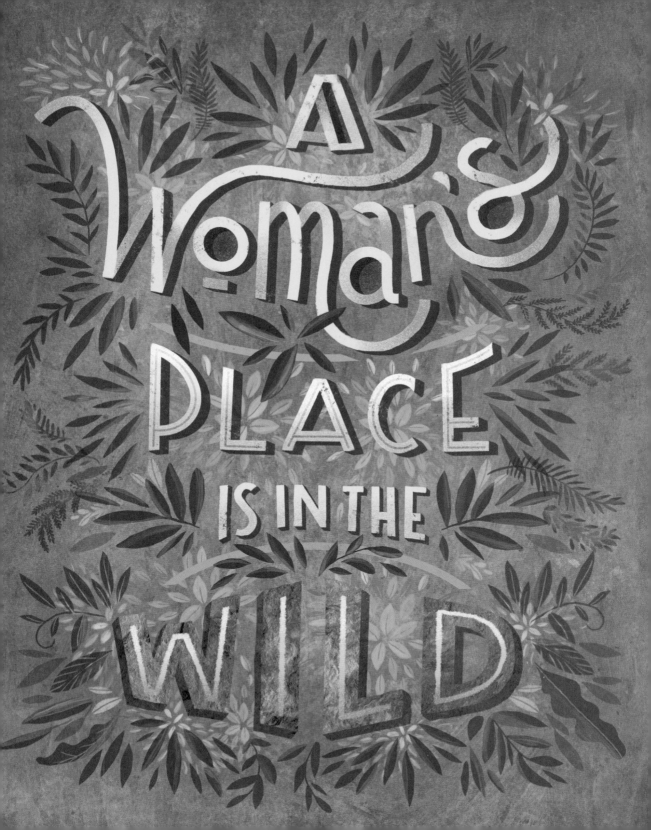

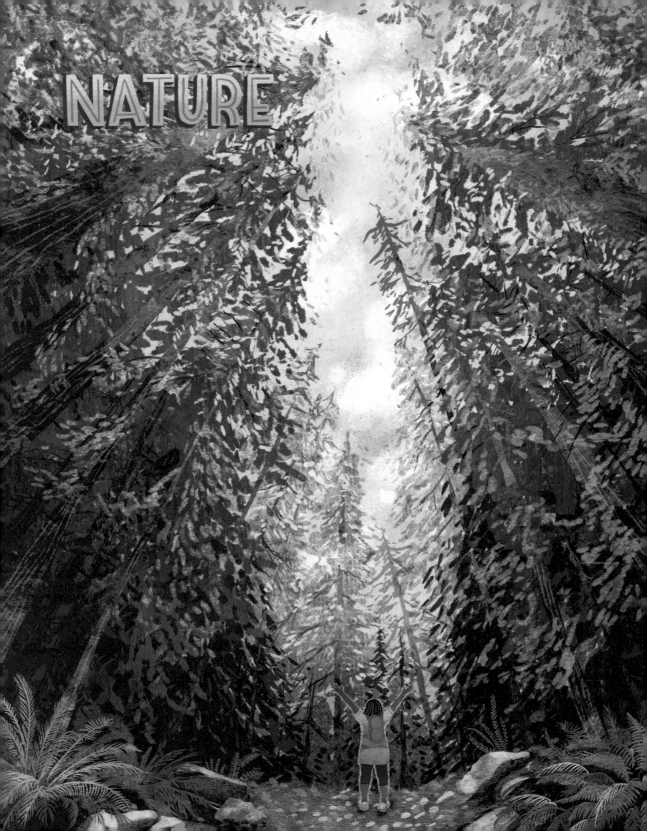

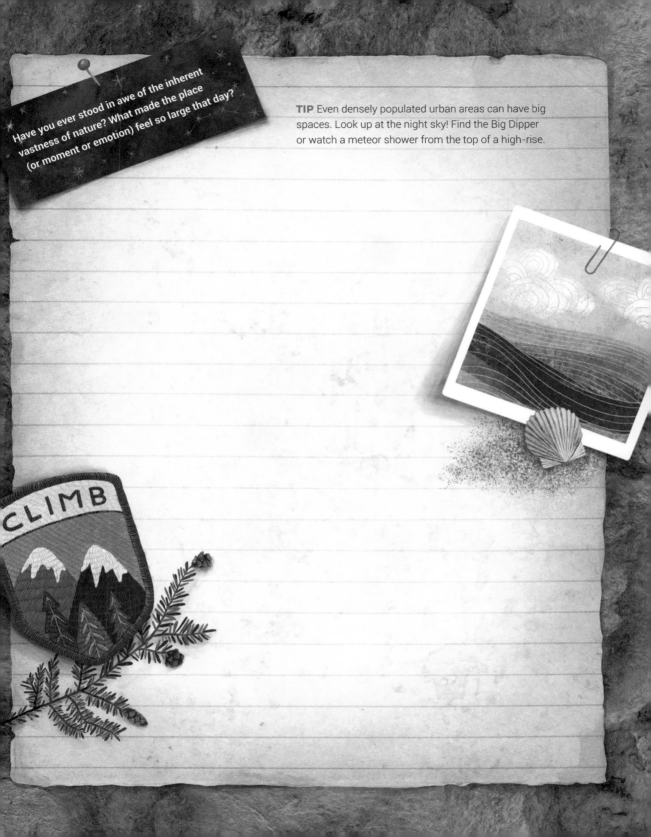

Have you ever stood in awe of the inherent vastness of nature? What made the place (or moment or emotion) feel so large that day?

TIP Even densely populated urban areas can have big spaces. Look up at the night sky! Find the Big Dipper or watch a meteor shower from the top of a high-rise.

CLIMB

SEE WITH YOUR FIVE SENSES

The "vastness of nature" exists in smaller places or daily moments that we often take for granted—the mix of scents in a garden, a full moon casting light on your upturned face, a cricket chirping in your backyard. Step outside and listen and look carefully. What do you hear? The buzzing of bees or of distant traffic? How does the grass feel beneath your bare feet, and how does the air smell? How many shades of green can you see?

Using all five senses, describe your surroundings in detail:

_____

_____

_____

_____

_____

_____

_____

_____

_____

_____

_____

_____

_____

_____

_____

_____

_____

_____

_____

_____

_____

_____

OBSERVE SLOWLY

Find a comfortable spot outside where you can sit for a while with some colored pencils or paints and paper. Watch and make notes or color swatches of all the things around you—trees, flowers, birds, insects, clouds. As you watch over time, how does the light shift in the trees? How does the color of the sky change? How does seeing a butterfly or bird affect your mood? The more you notice in your time spent outside, the more you will appreciate your outdoor adventures.

8:50 AM

12:50 PM

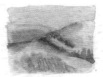

2:50 PM

6:45 PM SUNSET

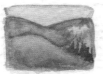

7:20 PM

8:45 PM

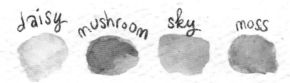

daisy   mushroom   sky   moss

NATURE'S TREASURE HUNT

For a fun challenge, head outside and see what catches your eye—a tiny leaf, an acorn, an unusual rock? Gather your treasures and sketch or paint them. Look at your objects from all angles. The goal is not to create a perfect piece of art but to train your eye to see each exquisite detail and notice any patterns or shifts in color with the light. Even a simple color swatch can capture the essence of a flower, spider, or pine cone. Fill this space with beauty:

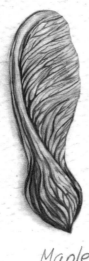

Maple Seed

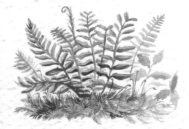

WILD FERN ON MOSS

Wing found on the way to the cascades

seed pod

driftwood

Treat future outings like this first treasure hunt.
Take in the subtle details of the natural world around you.

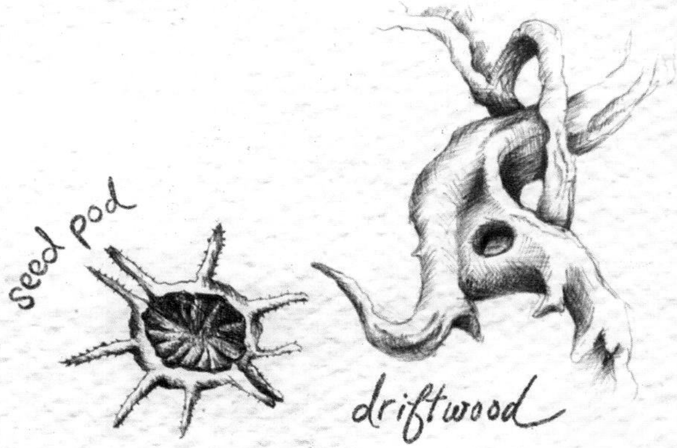

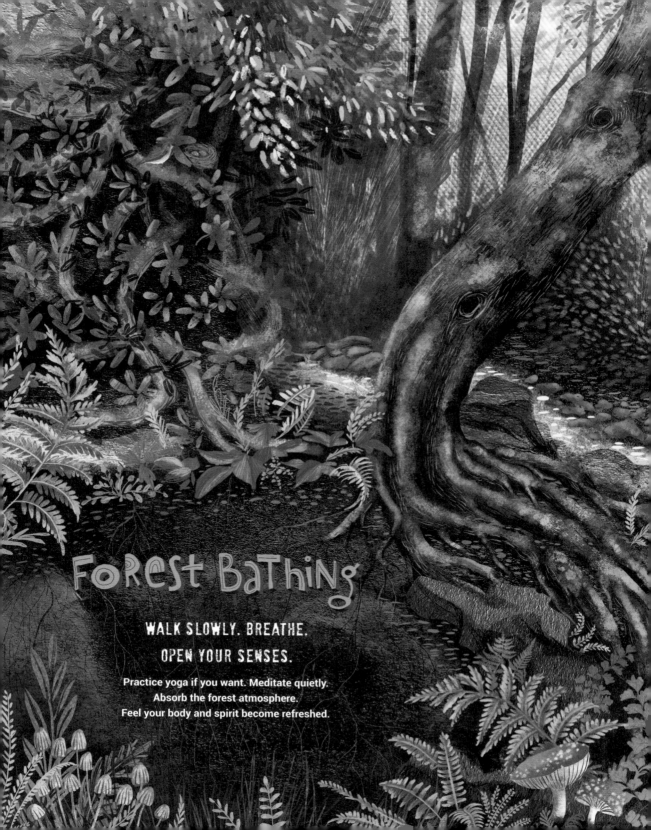

FOREST BATHING

WALK SLOWLY. BREATHE.
OPEN YOUR SENSES.

Practice yoga if you want. Meditate quietly.
Absorb the forest atmosphere.
Feel your body and spirit become refreshed.

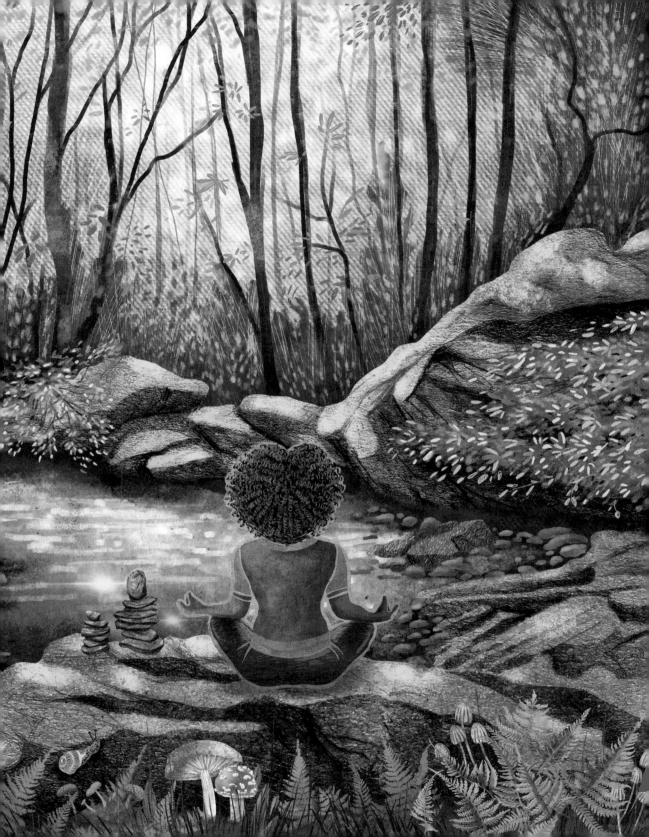

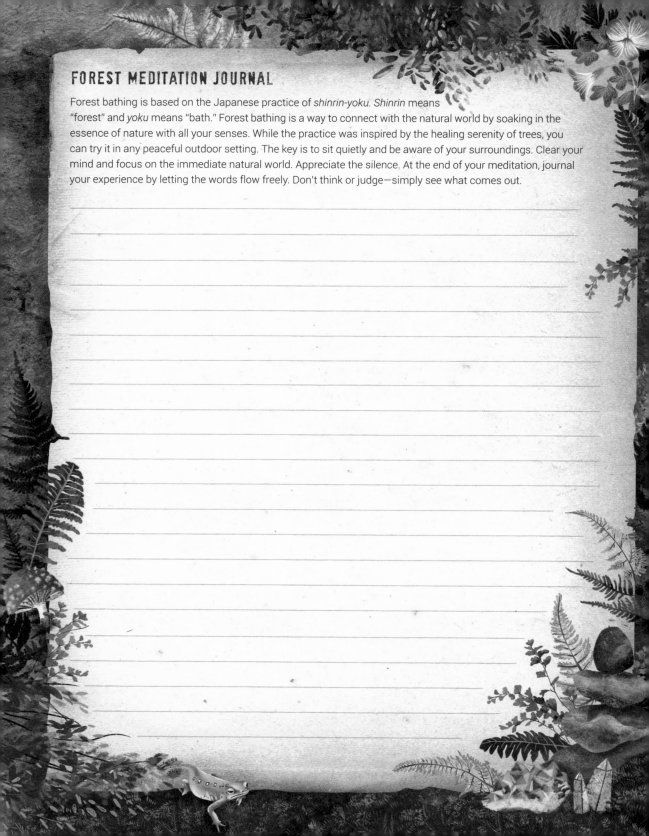

FOREST MEDITATION JOURNAL

Forest bathing is based on the Japanese practice of *shinrin-yoku*. *Shinrin* means "forest" and *yoku* means "bath." Forest bathing is a way to connect with the natural world by soaking in the essence of nature with all your senses. While the practice was inspired by the healing serenity of trees, you can try it in any peaceful outdoor setting. The key is to sit quietly and be aware of your surroundings. Clear your mind and focus on the immediate natural world. Appreciate the silence. At the end of your meditation, journal your experience by letting the words flow freely. Don't think or judge—simply see what comes out.

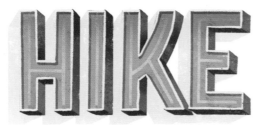

HIKE

REGULAR PEOPLE DO AMAZING THINGS ALL THE TIME. FIND SOMETHING THAT INTRIGUES YOU AND THAT YOU ARE HAPPY DOING. THEN BEGIN—NO EXPECTATIONS.

When I was a child, I spent entire days running barefoot in the grass, exploring the woods alone, catching crawfish in the creek, and hunting for fossils until the fireflies at dusk alerted me it was time for dinner. Adult responsibilities pulled me away from those magical summers . . . until I found my way back to nature and the outdoors through hiking. It's such a simple way to begin, and most places, even urban areas, have walking trails. I find many hikers and trekkers inspiring, not just because they have accomplished big adventures but because they are regular people who remind us that we can have extraordinary experiences with a little effort and planning.

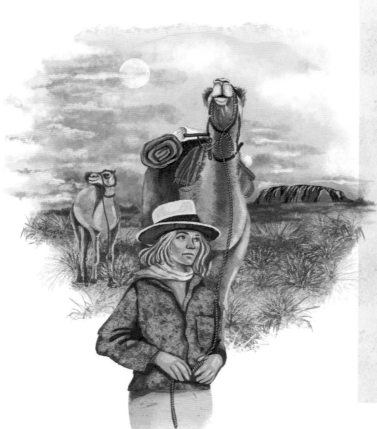

ROBYN DAVIDSON

THE "CAMEL LADY"

Robyn Davidson set off in 1977, at the age of twenty-seven, to walk 1,700 miles alone across the deserts of Western Australian with her dog and four camels she had trained for the adventure. Having no previous experience, she worked hard to gain the skills necessary to survive the harsh environment and reach the Pacific Ocean. Her book *Tracks* is an inspiring account of that journey.

More than four decades after her Outback crossing, Davidson described what she hopes her lasting legacy will be: "You can expand your boundaries; you don't have to obey the rules. You can experiment with your life in all sorts of ways. . . . Don't be so tied in by society's rules or your own inner rules."

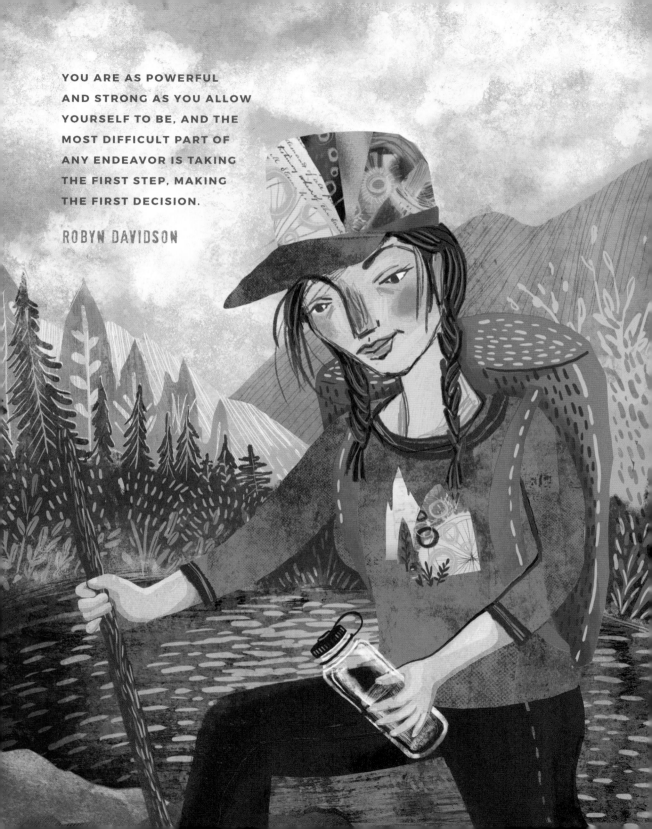

YOU ARE AS POWERFUL
AND STRONG AS YOU ALLOW
YOURSELF TO BE, AND THE
MOST DIFFICULT PART OF
ANY ENDEAVOR IS TAKING
THE FIRST STEP, MAKING
THE FIRST DECISION.

ROBYN DAVIDSON

TRIP PLANNING

No matter the adventure, even if it's just a short day hike, always let someone know where you are going, who you are going with, and when you plan to return. Before every trip, check the weather forecast and trail conditions and make sure you have the supplies you need. Even seasoned adventurers get caught in bad weather or have accidents. Bottom line: **Be prepared!**

Before you leave, text or email your trip plan to a trusted family member or friend. Here are two samples:

TRIP PLAN FOR A DAY HIKE

Name/Sex/Age

Address

Phone number

Car info

Start location, date, and time

End location and projected date and time

ITINERARY: List trail names and your destination(s).

TRIP PLAN FOR A MULTIDAY HIKE

Name/Sex/Age

Phone number

Address

Other members of party (names and phone numbers)

Car info

Existing medical problems and medications

Your gear (tent color, outerwear color, number of days of food)

End location and projected date and time

Start location, date, and time

ITINERARY: List trail names, campsites, a backup plan, etc. A targeted search effort improves your chances.

If I do not return by _____ (date/time), please call 911 or _____ (ranger station/local rescue agency)

for _____ (the area where you're going).

Once you are back in cell range, call or text your contact to let them know you've completed your hike.

LEAVE NO TRACE

Imagine admiring a gorgeous vista only to look down and see bar wrappers, an apple core, or toilet paper scattered on the ground. It is far too easy to have a negative effect on natural areas. While many people know to avoid certain obvious behaviors, other seemingly innocent actions can be quite harmful, especially in popular or ecologically fragile destinations. The seven principles developed by the Leave No Trace Center for Outdoor Ethics serve as a framework for minimizing your impact in the outdoors. Learn more about the principles at lnt.org.

PLAN AHEAD AND PREPARE

Research the area and regulations before you go. Make sure your group size is appropriate to ensure minimal impact. Repackage your food into resealable bags to reduce garbage. Small pieces of packaging are especially easy to drop.

TRAVEL AND CAMP ON DURABLE SURFACES

Camp on a durable surface such as rock, sand, or gravel instead of an area covered in fragile vegetation. Look for previously used campsites, and always sleep off the trail and at least 200 feet from any water sources.

Similarly, stick to clearly marked trails. As tempting as it may be to veer off the path to get a fantastic shot of yourself in that field of wildflowers, know that it can mark the way for other hikers to do the same. It doesn't take many boots to forever change the landscape.

DISPOSE OF WASTE PROPERLY

"Pack it in, pack it out" is your mantra. Litter is not just unsightly, it can be deadly. An orange or banana peel tossed into the woods with the thought that it's organic and will decompose is a big no-no. Those tasty scraps can attract animals, such as bears. And once animals begin to associate humans with food, they lose their fear of people and can become problematic—"problem" animals are often killed to protect humans. Don't be that person. (See "Wilderness Hygiene" for tips on how to dispose of human waste.)

LEAVE IT AS YOU FOUND IT

"Take nothing but pictures and kill nothing but time" is a great way to experience nature. Admire the flowers instead of picking them. Don't carve your name into a tree or bring a cultural artifact home as a souvenir.

MINIMIZE CAMPFIRE IMPACTS

Lightweight camp stoves have the least impact in the backcountry. If you hope to build a campfire, check the current fire danger level for your location and make sure there is not a burn ban in effect. If you do build a fire, use an existing fire ring, and do not bring wood from home: it can introduce pests into the area. Instead, collect dead wood locally to burn. After burning the wood to white ash, extinguish your fire completely and then spread out the ashes.

RESPECT WILDLIFE

Travel quietly and enjoy wildlife from afar. Do not attempt to get close for a photo, force creatures to flee, or try to feed them. If you see an injured animal, keep your distance and notify the game warden or ranger. Remember, we are visitors in their home.

BE CONSIDERATE OF OTHER VISITORS

Don't play loud music, bring pets that you cannot control, or do anything else to disturb the solitude for everyone. Land stewardship falls on each of us; by acting with respect, collectively we will keep the outdoors wild and beautiful.

DAY HIKING

Whether you're just getting started in the outdoors or training for bigger adventures, day hiking is an easy way to spend more time in nature. Keep your hike relaxing and fun with these basic items of gear and essential supplies.

WHAT TO PACK

- **FOOTWEAR:** Boots, trail runners, or hiking sandals are your most important gear. Your toes need to have enough wiggle room so that they don't hit the fronts of your boots when you're hiking downhill.

- **SOCKS:** Doubling up your socks can help prevent blisters. Choose thin liner socks and wool outer socks to reduce friction against your skin.

- **MOLESKIN OR LEUKOTAPE:** Keep a few pieces in your first-aid kit to treat or prevent blisters. See "Foot Care" for more.

- **LIGHTWEIGHT PACK:** Choose a day pack that comfortably fits the length of your back.

- **TREKKING POLES:** Not only do poles keep you steady, they reduce stress on your back and knees.

- **QUICK-DRY PANTS OR SHORTS:** Never wear denim or other forms of cotton. Cotton becomes heavy when wet, does not breathe, takes a long time to dry, and can cause hypothermia quickly if the temperature drops. The saying "cotton kills" exists for a reason.

- **HYDRATION:** Carry water bottles, or try a reservoir or bladder with a hose for hands-free hiking.

- **FOOD:** Bring healthy snacks such as fruit and nuts. Pack a little extra for emergencies.

- **THE TEN ESSENTIALS:** See "Backpacking" later for the full list. Assemble a small kit of these basics for a day out on the trail.

GET THE MOST OUT OF YOUR HIKE

1. **FIND AND RESEARCH GREAT LOCAL DAY HIKES. START WITH THESE RESOURCES:**
   - Apps such as AllTrails that provide GPS maps, current trail conditions, and reviews from fellow hikers
   - Guidebooks by local experts
   - Hiking groups organized by your local outfitter, a gear shop, or online through Meetup or other groups
   - Local organizations focused on hiking

2. **HIKE WITH FRIENDS.** Getting out in nature with friends, without the distraction of technology, is a fantastic way to connect on a deeper level and share amazing experiences you'll talk about for years to come.

3. **HIKE SOLO.** Making space for your thoughts away from others can be empowering and peaceful. Years ago while going through my divorce, I turned solo hiking into a walking meditation. You can heal your heart by concentrating on forward motion. Place one foot in front of the other and breathe deeply—your mind will clear.

4. **JOURNAL.** Carry a small notebook to record your hiking experiences. Journal your thoughts or simply take notes about the trail for future reference.

FUN TIP Add sketches to your notes when you stop for a break. Pack a travel-sized watercolor kit and paint with water from a stream to create a unique log of your outdoor journeys.

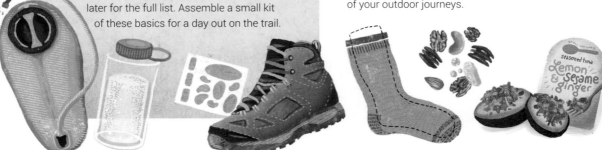

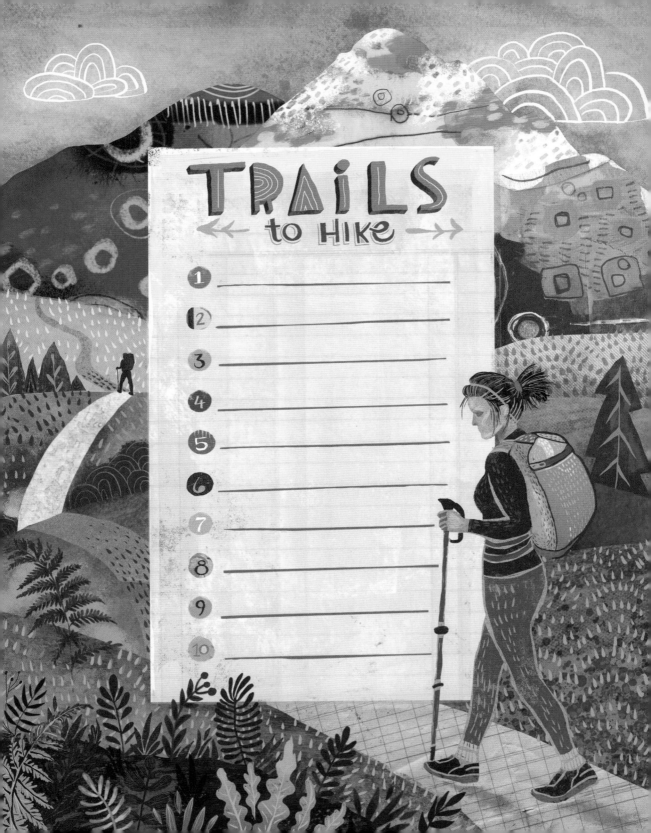

TRAILS
to Hike

1. _____
2. _____
3. _____
4. _____
5. _____
6. _____
7. _____
8. _____
9. _____
10. _____

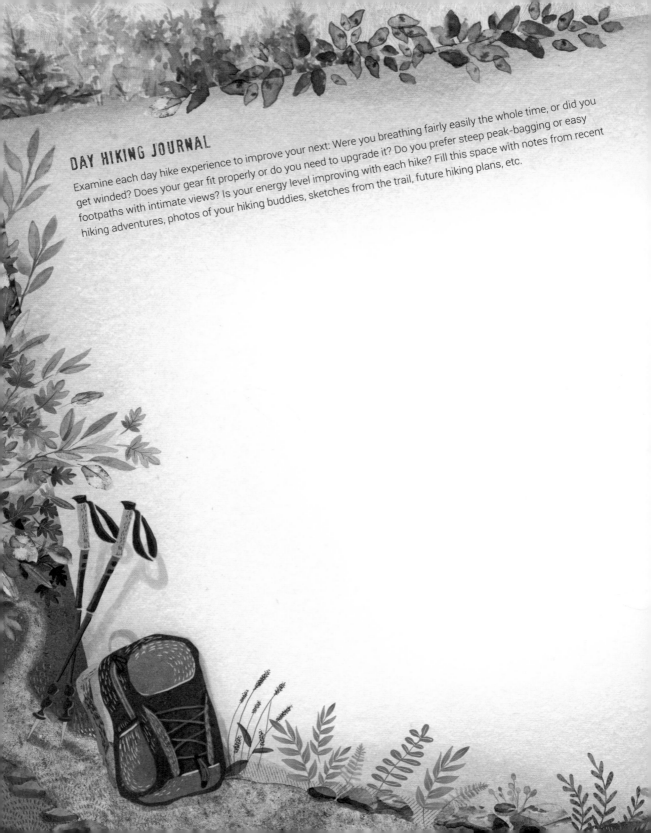

DAY HIKING JOURNAL

Examine each day hike experience to improve your next: Were you breathing fairly easily the whole time, or did you get winded? Does your gear fit properly or do you need to upgrade it? Do you prefer steep peak-bagging or easy footpaths with intimate views? Is your energy level improving with each hike? Fill this space with notes from recent hiking adventures, photos of your hiking buddies, sketches from the trail, future hiking plans, etc.

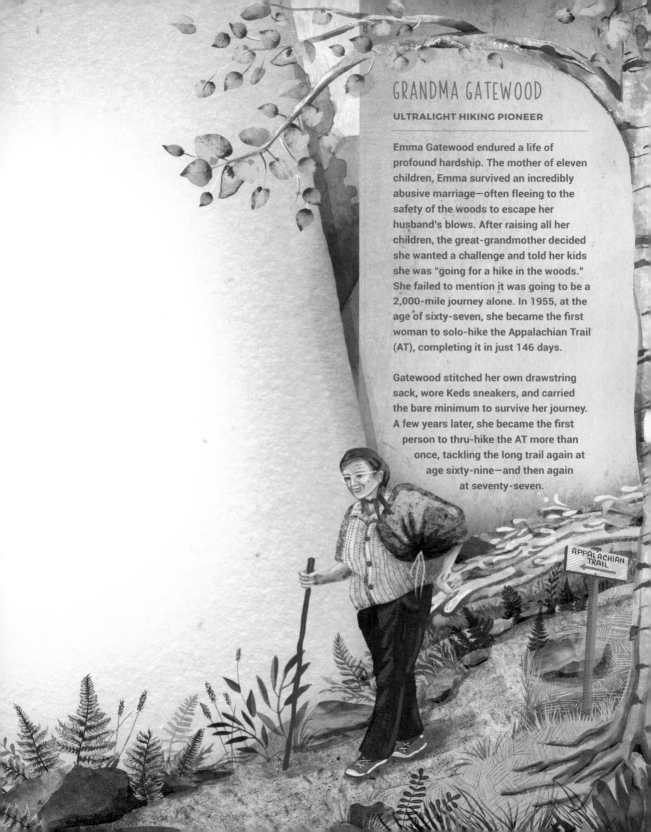

GRANDMA GATEWOOD

ULTRALIGHT HIKING PIONEER

Emma Gatewood endured a life of profound hardship. The mother of eleven children, Emma survived an incredibly abusive marriage—often fleeing to the safety of the woods to escape her husband's blows. After raising all her children, the great-grandmother decided she wanted a challenge and told her kids she was "going for a hike in the woods." She failed to mention it was going to be a 2,000-mile journey alone. In 1955, at the age of sixty-seven, she became the first woman to solo-hike the Appalachian Trail (AT), completing it in just 146 days.

Gatewood stitched her own drawstring sack, wore Keds sneakers, and carried the bare minimum to survive her journey. A few years later, she became the first person to thru-hike the AT more than once, tackling the long trail again at age sixty-nine—and then again at seventy-seven.

APPALACHIAN TRAIL

BACKPACKING

Think of backpacking as day hiking, but with everything you need on your back for a fully immersed outdoor adventure. Start with an overnight outing on a short trail close to home to test your gear. Soon you'll be planning multinight trips into the backcountry and low-key weekends in the woods with friends.

HOW TO LOAD A PACK

Customize this guide for your trip and your pack. Will you be checking it to fly to your destination? Put it in a secondhand duffel bag to protect the straps and buckles. Give away the duffel or mail it home once you've arrived if you don't need it for the trip home.

OUTER POCKET

Keep your maps, guides, first-aid kit, and snacks handy.

SIDE POCKETS

Stash your water bottles, filter, and fuel bottles (upright). If you'll be flying, you'll need to buy fuel at your destination.

SEPARATE LOWER COMPARTMENT

Some packs have a compartment for lighter gear: sleeping bag, tent footprint or tarp, hammock, camp chair, or sleeping pad. Most have bottom straps to lash some items to the outside.

TOP COMPARTMENT

Store items you want easy access to, such as raingear, headlamp, compass, sunscreen, knife, and snacks, in the top pocket.

RESERVOIR SLEEVE

This special feature close to your back is designed for a water bladder.

MIDDLE OF PACK

Pack heavy items, such as food, charging blocks, and cooking equipment, in the middle and close to your back, near your center of gravity.

HIP BELT POCKETS

These pockets are perfect for snacks, camera, GPS device, lip balm.

TIPS Store clothing and other essentials in waterproof stuff sacks or trash bags. Also, wrap some duct tape around your sunscreen tube, lighter, water bottle, or trekking poles for patching gear or making an emergency bandage.

BACKPACKING CHECKLIST

Use this handy list so you don't forget anything important. Customize it for the terrain, weather conditions, and length of your adventure.

- [ ] **SHELTER:** Tent (with footprint and rainfly), tarp, hammock, or bivy sack

- [ ] **SLEEP SYSTEM:** Sleeping bag and stuff sack, liner, pad

- [ ] **FOOD:** Meals, snacks, condiments, spices, oil, bear canister if in bear country

- [ ] **COOKING GEAR:** Stove, fuel, windscreen, pot with lifter, cup, bowl, utensil, camp soap

- [ ] **CLOTHING:** Socks, underwear, sports bra, pants, shirt, leggings, shorts or skirt, base layers, long-sleeve shirt, warm jacket, gloves, hat, raingear, camp shoes

- [ ] **BATHROOM:** Toilet paper, trowel, hand sanitizer, baby wipes, menstrual products, sealable plastic bags to pack out trash

- [ ] **TOILETRIES:** Toothbrush and paste, soap, contacts and glasses, comb, mirror, hair ties, foot salve, prescription medications

- [ ] **THE TEN ESSENTIALS:** See list at right. Also: insect repellent, whistle, solar inflatable light, nylon cord

- [ ] **COMMUNICATION:** Cell phone, charging block, PLB (personal locator beacon) or GPS device/satellite communicator

- [ ] **DON'T FORGET:** Permits, keys, cash and/or credit cards, driver's license, important phone numbers

THE TEN ESSENTIALS

Customize this iconic survival list of baseline gear, developed by The Mountaineers, for each adventure. Put together a small essentials kit in a waterproof bag for day trips. For longer treks or more extreme conditions, tailor each item to the location and expected weather. The goal is to be prepared to respond to an emergency and safely spend an unexpected night outside.

1. **NAVIGATION:** Maps, compass, altimeter watch, GPS device

2. **HEADLAMP:** A hands-free light source plus extra batteries

3. **SUN PROTECTION:** Sunscreen, hat, sunglasses, lip balm, sun-protective clothing

4. **FIRST AID:** Compact kit containing blister treatment, bandages, gauze, tape, a wrap, disinfecting ointment, gloves, tweezers, a needle, antihistamine and antidiarrheal medicine, topical antibiotic cream, over-the-counter pain relievers, EpiPen (if your allergies require it), and other personal medications

5. **KNIFE:** A multitool or pocketknife; plus repair items such as safety pins, wire, duct tape, zip ties, various replacement parts

6. **FIRE:** Lighter, waterproof matches, firestarter, tinder

7. **SHELTER:** Tent, emergency bivy sack, or space blanket; a large plastic trash bag is a cheap, light option: to prevent hypothermia in an emergency, punch a small breathing hole in a bottom corner and then crouch on the ground inside the bag in the driest nearby location

8. **NUTRITION:** An extra day's supply of food (or more for longer trips) in case of emergency

9. **HYDRATION:** Ample water (in bottles or bladders) and a water treatment system or tablets; for a desert environment, research water sources ahead of time

10. **EXTRA CLOTHES:** Additional base layers or other dry items for keeping your core warm

WILDERNESS HYGIENE

Whether you're out for a long day hike or spending a week in the woods, you'll want to be prepared, but also comfortable.

The 3 Ps! Pee, Poop, and Periods
These basic biological functions cause beginners quite a bit of anxiety, but once you learn a few tips, you'll no longer dread the inevitable . . . at least not as much.

Pee
Number one is easy!

- **Move 200 feet off the trail** or away from your campsite or water.

- **Verify the area is clear** of stinging nettles, poison oak, or other problematic plants.

- **Squat, pee, and then shake it off or wipe** using toilet paper, a bandanna, or a Kula Cloth. Whatever you use, pack it out. My leave-no-trace preference is the Kula Cloth, a reusable pee cloth—urine only!—with an antimicrobial absorbent side. Snap it to your pack to let it dry, then rinse it at home or camp.

- **Pee funnels enable you to go while standing up,** but they can be messy. If you want to use one on the trail, practice with it at home in the shower first.

Periods
Let's face it, periods are never fun to deal with—even less so in nature. But don't let your monthly cycle deter you from spending time outdoors.

- **Try a lightweight, reusable menstrual cup** to eliminate trash on the trail. Practice using it before your trip to make sure it's a good fit. Once outside, empty the cup into a cat hole, rinse it with water, then reinsert it.

- If you prefer tampons (or pads), **choose a brand without an applicator** so you'll have less trash to pack out. Never put used tampons in a cat hole—animals might dig them up. Instead, pack them out in a separate zip-top bag.

- **Always keep one or two tampons in your pack.** Spending time outdoors can alter the timing of your cycle, and you don't want to be in the wilderness without protection.

Poop
When going number two, be careful to keep water sources free of pollution and camping zones clean.

- **Find an area at least 200 feet from any water, trails, and campsites** and where people are unlikely to walk.

- **Dig a cat hole six inches deep** with your trowel, preferably in dark, organic soil, which aids decomposition.

- **Squat over the hole, do your business, put the used TP** into a zip-top plastic bag, then cover the waste with dirt and organic matter. **TIP** Dig your cat hole beside a log so you can sit while you go—just like at home but with a better view!

- **Some high-traffic or fragile areas require everyone to pack out solid waste in a wag bag,** a sealable two-bag system with a powder that breaks down solids. Store the bags in your pack and toss them in the next trash can you come across.

Other Helpful Bathroom Tips
- **Hike with a plastic bag with clean wet wipes or tissue** and an empty zip-top bag for used products. If nature calls while you're on the go, you'll have everything you need within reach.

- **Rocks, moss, sticks, leaves (know your species!), and handfuls of snow make good TP alternatives.** The first time I tried snow, it took my breath away, but now it is my favorite method in the backcountry.

- For longer trips where pack weight is critical, **remove the cardboard roll from your TP and dry out your pack of baby wipes.** You can easily rehydrate them on the trail—good as new!

Foot Care

No matter how much TLC you give your feet, they are going to take a beating on the trail. Something as small as a blister can ruin an otherwise amazing outing: treat or prevent them as soon as you feel a hotspot forming.

Here are some other ways you can protect your feet:

- **Make sure your shoes or boots fit you properly,** and break them in before your trip. Tighten your laces before hiking downhill to prevent rubbing.

- **Wear thin sock liners** underneath wool or synthetic-blend hiking socks.

- **Pack Leukotape, moleskin, gel pads, and other bandages** to cover any hotspots. **TIP** Reduce bulk by cutting small pieces of Leukotape off the roll and applying them to wax paper. Store in a baggie until needed.

- **Rub a soothing salve** on your feet at the end of the day.

- **Keep your feet dry.** Place damp socks (and other wet items) in your sleeping bag at night to dry them.

Chafing can happen elsewhere too. Apply an anti-chafe product as needed throughout the day, and change out of wet, sweaty clothes when setting up camp.

Brushing Your Teeth

Brush as you always do, but don't spit out your toothpaste in one large glob. Instead, sip some water and then spew the diluted toothpaste in a diffuse spray over some bushes or the ground. The idea is to make it less concentrated to protect animals in case they ingest it.

Bathing

Want to stay extra-clean on the trail? Bring a compact backpacking shower, a bag with a nozzle that you can fill and then suspend from a tree. If you're hiking and camping near lakes and rivers, take a dip instead—a welcome treat on a hot day. Either way, always use biodegradable soap! Unscented baby wipes can also freshen you up in a pinch, but be sure to pack them out.

TIP Leave the scented products at home, especially if you're going to be traveling in bear country.

BACKPACKING JOURNAL

Describe a trip you never want to forget. Did you meet any unusual or intriguing people along the trail? Keep track of the trail wisdom, tips, and hacks you've learned so your next backpacking adventure will be even better.

TRAIL TALK

Even if you're not planning a thru-hike on a destination trail, it's still fun to learn the lingo.

THRU-HIKE: An end-to-end hike on a long-distance trail within twelve months

SECTION-HIKE: Hiking a longer trail in shorter sections

LASH (long-ass section hiker): Someone who section-hikes for weeks or months at a time

FLIP-FLOP: To hike a full trail from the middle and complete it in sections nonsequentially, often to avoid bad weather

NOBO: Northbound on a trail

SOBO: Southbound on a trail

TRAIL MAGIC: When trail "angels" spontaneously show up with food, drinks, supplies, or a free ride

WHITE BLAZES: Trail markers found on trees along the Appalachian Trail

BLUE BLAZES: Markers along the AT indicating a spur trail to a water source or a great view

YELLOW BLAZES: The yellow lines on a highway, meaning you hitchhiked or drove to skip parts of a trail; prepare to catch flak from your fellow hikers

PINK OR DUDE BLAZING: When a hiker pursues a potential love interest on the trail

TRAMILY: Your trail family that you make along the way

SLACK-PACKING: Hiking with basics like food and water while your gear is shuttled ahead of you

TAKE A ZERO: A rest day

PUDS: Pointless ups and downs

VITAMIN I: Ibuprofen

MIDRANGE AND LONG-DISTANCE TRAILS

Once you have some shorter backpacking trips under your belt, consider working your way up to greater distances. Tackling one of the following midrange trails is great preparation for a longer thru-hike, such as the Pacific Crest Trail, Appalachian Trail, or Continental Divide Trail. If you don't have four or five months to do a thru-hike, try section-hiking a long trail instead. That way you can knock off 30-to-50-mile segments over a week or ten days!

TRAILS TO DREAM ABOUT

Grand Canyon Rim-to-Rim Hike, Arizona (24 miles)

Four Pass Loop, Colorado (28 miles)

Inca Trail (26 miles), **Lares Trek** (21 miles), and **Salkantay Trail** (46 miles), **Peru**

Timberline Trail, Oregon (41 miles)

W Trek, Patagonia, Chile (46 miles)

Hadrian's Wall Path, England (84 miles)

Wonderland Trail, Washington (93 miles)

John Muir Trail, California (211 miles)

Via Transilvanica, Romania (590 miles)

HUT-TO-HUT TRAILS

Try a different kind of backcountry trek that involves hiking between rustic shelters—a yurt, cabin, teahouse, *albergue*, or off-the-grid hotel. Hut-based routes are very popular in Europe, but there are also many options in North America.

A FEW HUT CIRCUITS TO TRY

San Juan Huts, Colorado (4.5 to 8.5 miles apart)

White Mountain Huts, New Hampshire (6 to 8 miles apart)

High Sierra Camps, California (49 miles)

Laugavegur Trail, Iceland (34 miles)

Tour du Mont Blanc, Europe (110 miles)

Annapurna Circuit, Nepal (128 miles)

Camino de Santiago, Camino Francés, France and Spain (500 miles)

BACKPACKING TRAILS I HOPE TO HIKE

NAME / LOCATION	DIFFICULTY	DISTANCE

GET THE MOST OUT OF YOUR BACKCOUNTRY TRAIL TIME

Trail wisdom warns, "Don't pack your fears." In other words, don't bring all the things you *might* need. There is nothing worse than being overloaded, in pain, and miserable. Always pack the essentials, but do you really need all those changes of clothes? Can't your mug be your bowl as well? On the other hand, certain luxury items are well worth their extra weight. I like to carry a travel watercolor kit and loose paper for sketching at camp. You may want to bring a book, harmonica, binoculars, or deck of cards.

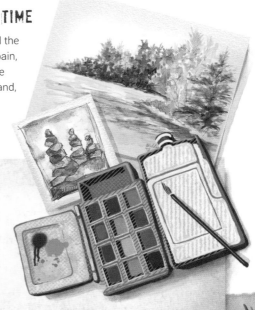

What's the most ridiculous thing you've regretted putting in your pack?

What are your must-have luxury items?

THE TRIPLE CROWN

Drawing thousands of people each year, these three premier routes rank high among the eleven National Scenic Trails designated by the National Park System. Hikers who walk each footpath in its entirety will have covered nearly 8,000 miles and can add the title "Triple Crowner" to their list of accomplishments.

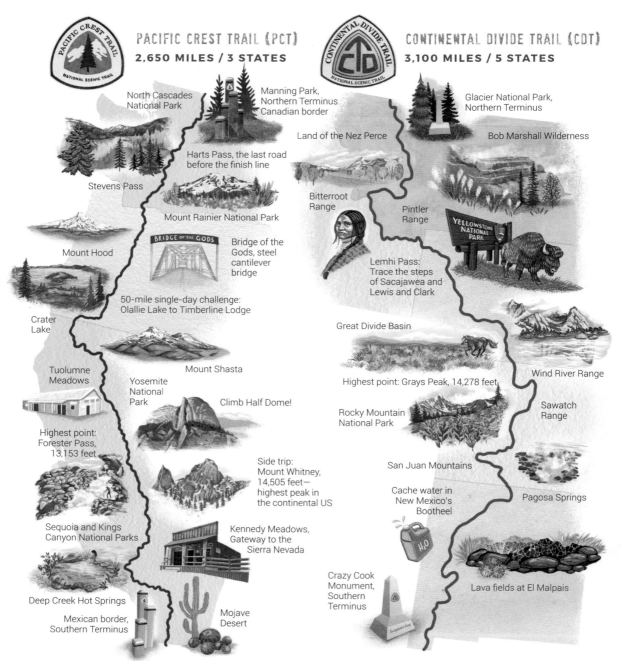

PACIFIC CREST TRAIL (PCT)
2,650 MILES / 3 STATES

- North Cascades National Park
- Manning Park, Northern Terminus Canadian border
- Harts Pass, the last road before the finish line
- Stevens Pass
- Mount Rainier National Park
- Mount Hood
- Bridge of the Gods, steel cantilever bridge
- 50-mile single-day challenge: Olallie Lake to Timberline Lodge
- Crater Lake
- Mount Shasta
- Tuolumne Meadows
- Yosemite National Park
- Climb Half Dome!
- Highest point: Forester Pass, 13,153 feet
- Side trip: Mount Whitney, 14,505 feet—highest peak in the continental US
- Sequoia and Kings Canyon National Parks
- Kennedy Meadows, Gateway to the Sierra Nevada
- Deep Creek Hot Springs
- Mojave Desert
- Mexican border, Southern Terminus

CONTINENTAL DIVIDE TRAIL (CDT)
3,100 MILES / 5 STATES

- Glacier National Park, Northern Terminus
- Land of the Nez Perce
- Bob Marshall Wilderness
- Bitterroot Range
- Pintler Range
- Yellowstone National Park
- Lemhi Pass: Trace the steps of Sacajawea and Lewis and Clark
- Great Divide Basin
- Wind River Range
- Highest point: Grays Peak, 14,278 feet
- Rocky Mountain National Park
- Sawatch Range
- San Juan Mountains
- Cache water in New Mexico's Bootheel
- Pagosa Springs
- Lava fields at El Malpais
- Crazy Cook Monument, Southern Terminus

HiKe YOUR OWN HiKe — NEVER QUIT ON A BAD DAY

Do what is best for you and at your own pace.

APPALACHIAN TRAIL (AT)
2,190 MILES / 14 STATES

APPALACHIAN TRAIL — NATIONAL SCENIC TRAIL

Mount Katahdin, Northern Terminus

Saddleback Mountain

100 Mile Wilderness — a remote, nearly inaccessible forest

TIP Most hikers use the Guthook Guides app to get current, crowdsourced trail conditions and water reports.

Mount Greylock

Pine Grove Furnace State Park: Take the half-gallon ice cream challenge

White Mountains

Mount Washington, longtime record for fastest recorded wind speed: 231 mph

Ice Cream — HALF WAY!

Historic Harpers Ferry

McAfee Knob

Shenandoah National Park

Dragons Tooth

Great Smoky Mountains, most-visited US national park

Cherokee National Forest

Clingmans Dome, highest point at 6,643 feet

Charlies Bunion

Neels Gap, legendary gear shakedown at Mountain Crossings outfitter

Springer Mountain, Southern Terminus

HEATHER "ANISH" ANDERSON

TRIPLE CROWN TRAILBLAZER

Heather Anderson, known as Anish on trails, wasn't always athletic. In her first memoir *Thirst: 2600 Miles to Home* she recalls being a quiet, overweight kid who retreated into the world of books. Her love of hiking began when she spent a summer in college working in the Grand Canyon. On her first backpacking trip, she hiked the Grand Canyon Rim-to-Rim route with borrowed gear and feet protected only by duct tape after her sandals fell apart a few miles in.

Anish went on to hike the Appalachian Trail, Pacific Crest Trail, and Continental Divide Trail— the Triple Crown—and later set speed records for self-supported hikes of the AT and PCT. In 2018 the National Geographic Adventurer of the Year hiked all three trails again, this time in a single calendar year, specifically 251 days, 20 hours, and 10 minutes, becoming the first woman to accomplish this impressive athletic feat. As she explains in *Mud, Rocks, Blazes*, her memoir of her record-setting AT hike, "The trail has a way of answering the questions you most need answered, even if you are afraid to ask."

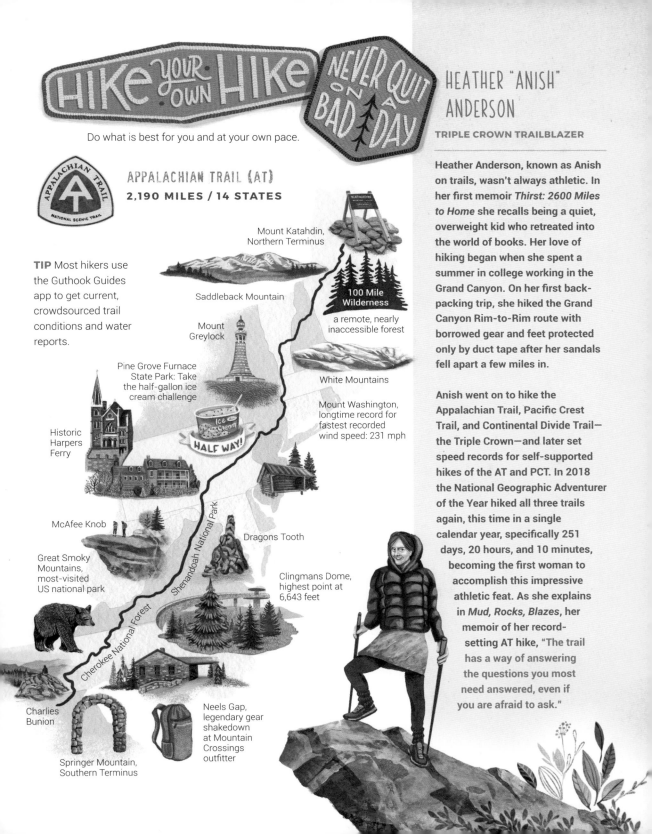

MIRNA VALERIO

**ULTRAMARATHON RUNNER
—THE MIRNAVATOR**

National Geographic named Mirna Valerio an Adventurer of the Year for her ground-breaking work challenging the stereotype of what a runner should look like. First on her blog *Fat Girl Running* and now on her website themirnavator.com, Valerio tackles body shaming while educating others to start where they already are, physically and mentally. "Fit comes in many forms and people can still participate in athletics no matter what kind of body they have."

An advocate for more diverse represen-tations in social media, Valerio wants everyone to have a "really deep, profound experience with nature that you can't have looking out a window." You can find her in a 50K race, on a 120-mile run, or doing yoga by a stream, all while breaking cultural norms. This is what an athlete looks like.

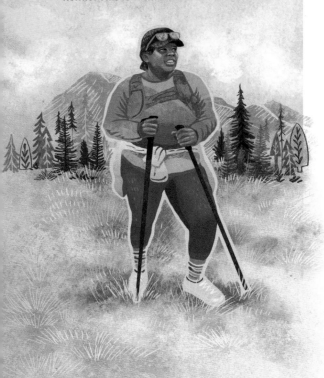

RUN

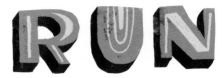

Running is a great way to squeeze outdoor exercise into a busy workday or between errands. But it can also become a way of life, taking you to amazing cities or into the wilderness on mountain trails.

GETTING STARTED

Running well begins with great shoes—and a good warm-up.

Shoes: This is your most critical piece of gear. A gait analysis at your local running store will get you into the best pair for your foot-strike style and your goals.

Clothing: Wear items made of breathable, moisture-wicking material that are not too baggy and will not chafe. You'll also need a supportive sports bra, synthetic or wool running socks, and a hat. Carry your keys, phone, water, and snacks in pockets, an armband, a waist belt, or a running-specific hydration vest.

Couch to 5K: This well-known training program begins gently, alternating running for one minute with walking for two minutes. Over several weeks, you'll increase your running time and distance while building speed and endurance. Keep your motivation high with a GPS app like Runkeeper, which tracks your pace, time, route, and calories while offering encouraging prompts.

Other Tips:

• Try a dynamic warm-up of leg swings, arm swings, knee hugs, quad stretches, and lunges before each run to activate your muscles and reduce your risk of injury.

• Maintain an easy pace and take days off as your body adjusts.

• In the beginning, focus on running for a set amount of time instead of a certain speed or distance.

• Stay motivated by running with a buddy and adding variety: find new routes to explore and change up your running surfaces. If you look forward to each run, it will become a consistent habit.

ORGANIZED RUNS

Participate in an organized run to improve your skills, challenge yourself, and perhaps even raise money for a good cause. Find an event near you, or seek out a destination race. Track your race details here.

5KS

RACE	TIME

10KS

RACE	TIME

OBSTACLE COURSES

Test your mettle and get muddy with obstacle challenges such as Muddy Dash, Tough Mudder, Spartan Race, and Warrior Dash.

RACE	TIME

FUN RUNS

Even if you don't consider yourself a runner, nothing compares to the festival-like atmosphere of a fun run. Grab some friends and do a Foam Glow, a turkey trot, or the eccentric Bay to Breakers—or flee zombies in the Run for Your Lives race. You'll find some people jogging and others walking, so don't let your inexperience keep you away.

My son and I particularly love The Color Run race series, in which participants become human art canvases while running through clouds of colorful powder. If people-watching is your favorite sport, then a fun run is your Olympics. Find a crazy hat or outrageous costume and join them!

RACE / LOCATION

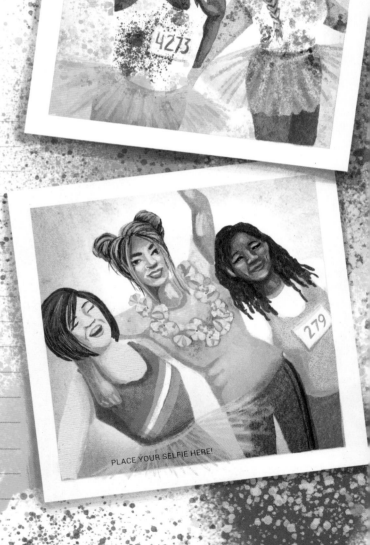

PLACE YOUR SELFIE HERE!

HALF-MARATHONS

Run a half-marathon as part of your training regimen for a full marathon, or choose a half at a fun destination for a "runcation" with friends.

RACE / LOCATION	TIME

MARATHONS

A 26.2-mile test of your training and endurance—this may be the ultimate running goal. Do you dream of qualifying for the iconic Boston Marathon? Or are you drawn to something more extreme like the North Pole Marathon or the Everest Marathon? Running one in every state would be epic, but completing even a single marathon is a tremendous accomplishment.

RACE / LOCATION	TIME

MAKE YOUR MARATHON TRAINING PLAN

Training for longer events can take months. Build up your mileage, pace, and strength slowly while listening to your body to avoid injury. Each week tackle one long run—extend the distance over time—and take at least one full rest day. On the other days, mix up short runs, yoga, easy jogging, and cross training. Every few weeks, reduce your overall volume for a week to allow your body to absorb the training and recover. Record your training runs below as you prepare. For a marathon, most sources recommend sixteen to eighteen weeks of training.

	SUN	MON	TUES	WED	THURS	FRI	SAT	TOTAL MILEAGE
1								
2								
3								
4								
5								
6								

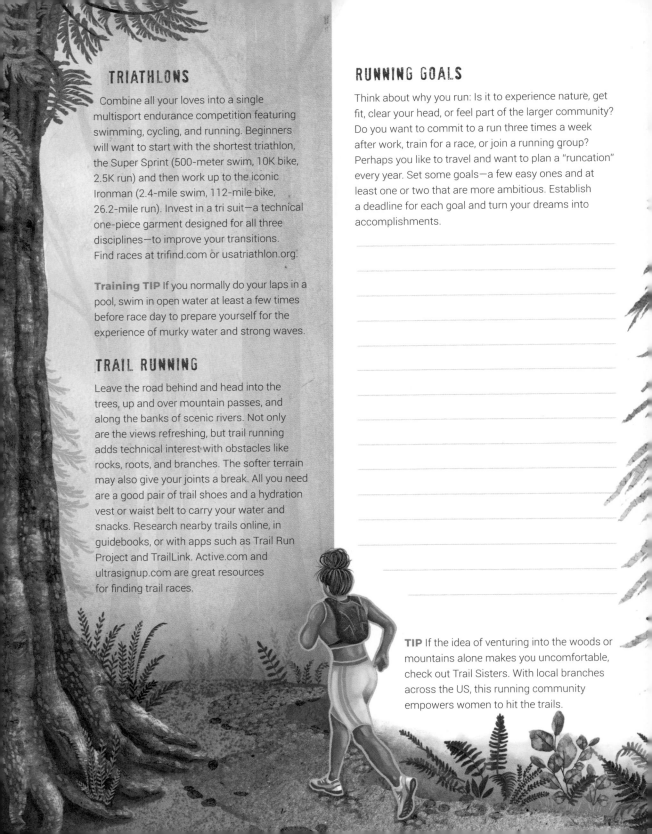

TRIATHLONS

Combine all your loves into a single multisport endurance competition featuring swimming, cycling, and running. Beginners will want to start with the shortest triathlon, the Super Sprint (500-meter swim, 10K bike, 2.5K run) and then work up to the iconic Ironman (2.4-mile swim, 112-mile bike, 26.2-mile run). Invest in a tri suit—a technical one-piece garment designed for all three disciplines—to improve your transitions. Find races at trifind.com or usatriathlon.org.

Training TIP If you normally do your laps in a pool, swim in open water at least a few times before race day to prepare yourself for the experience of murky water and strong waves.

TRAIL RUNNING

Leave the road behind and head into the trees, up and over mountain passes, and along the banks of scenic rivers. Not only are the views refreshing, but trail running adds technical interest with obstacles like rocks, roots, and branches. The softer terrain may also give your joints a break. All you need are a good pair of trail shoes and a hydration vest or waist belt to carry your water and snacks. Research nearby trails online, in guidebooks, or with apps such as Trail Run Project and TrailLink. Active.com and ultrasignup.com are great resources for finding trail races.

RUNNING GOALS

Think about why you run: Is it to experience nature, get fit, clear your head, or feel part of the larger community? Do you want to commit to a run three times a week after work, train for a race, or join a running group? Perhaps you like to travel and want to plan a "runcation" every year. Set some goals—a few easy ones and at least one or two that are more ambitious. Establish a deadline for each goal and turn your dreams into accomplishments.

TIP If the idea of venturing into the woods or mountains alone makes you uncomfortable, check out Trail Sisters. With local branches across the US, this running community empowers women to hit the trails.

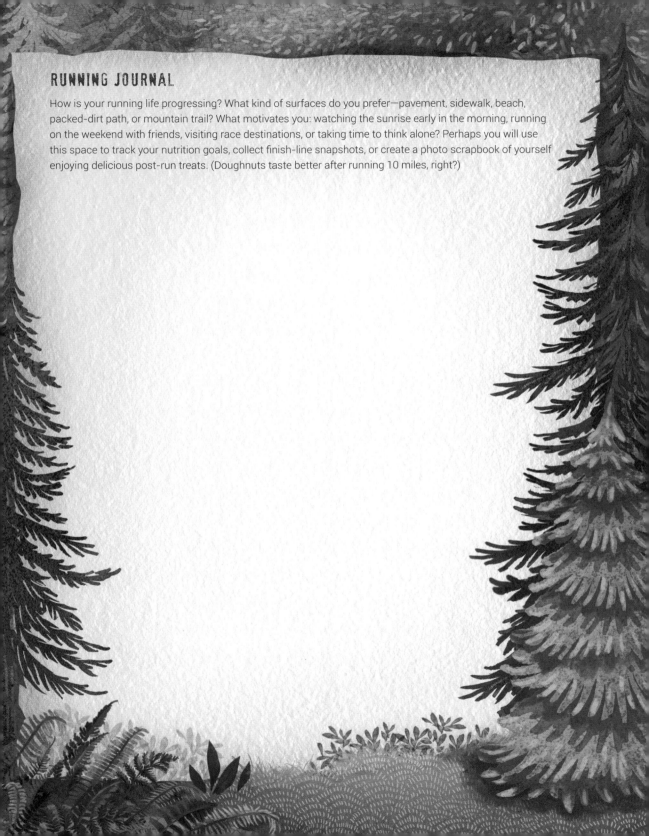

RUNNING JOURNAL

How is your running life progressing? What kind of surfaces do you prefer—pavement, sidewalk, beach, packed-dirt path, or mountain trail? What motivates you: watching the sunrise early in the morning, running on the weekend with friends, visiting race destinations, or taking time to think alone? Perhaps you will use this space to track your nutrition goals, collect finish-line snapshots, or create a photo scrapbook of yourself enjoying delicious post-run treats. (Doughnuts taste better after running 10 miles, right?)

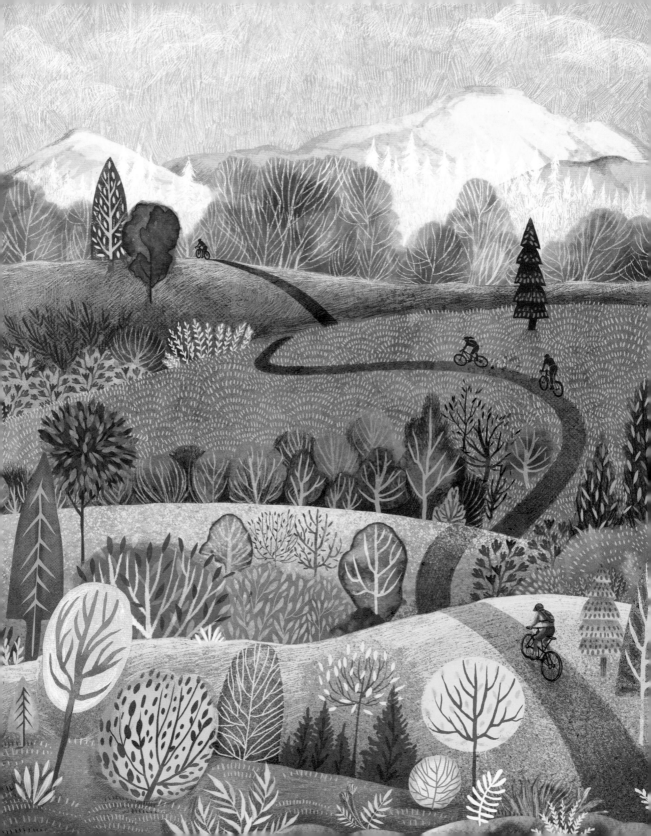

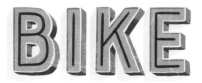

BIKE

I got my first taste of unrestricted freedom as a kid on my banana-seat bike with its colorful handlebar streamers. Roaming the neighborhood with my girl gang, stopping only to eat, unencumbered by rules or a schedule, is a lifestyle I *still* chase. Whether you like fat tires and dirt trails or multiple gears and smooth pavement, hop on two wheels and recapture your childhood spirit.

MOUNTAIN BIKING

Heavier bikes, thicker tires, roots, rocks, steep terrain, berms—mountain biking is high-adrenaline fun! In their off-season, a growing number of ski resorts are opening up their alpine slopes to mountain bikers. Ride the lift up for a ridgetop cruise before barreling down the mountainside.

Start a list of trails, gravel and dirt roads, and bike parks that you want to ride. (Check out the Trailforks app to see what's near you.) Work through it, one track at a time.

NAME / LOCATION	DISTANCE

REBECCA RUSCH

AWARD-WINNING ULTRA-ENDURANCE ATHLETE

This multidiscipline athlete has earned the nickname "Queen of Pain" for her extraordinary ability to push her physical and mental endurance limits. "Fear and pain are incredible teachers," she says. Rusch was already a champion in cross-country skiing, whitewater rafting, expedition racing, orienteering, and rock climbing when she started her mountain bike career at age thirty-eight. In 2016, she summited Kilimanjaro (19,340 feet) by bike, later describing it as "absolutely the hardest ride I've done in my life." A four-time winner of the Leadville 100 and six-time winner of the Dirty Kanza, she was inducted into the Mountain Bike Hall of Fame in 2019.

When not on her bike, Rusch works as a part-time firefighter and EMT, runs the Be Good Foundation, and organizes Rebecca's Private Idaho, a premier gravel event. "All these guys will go out hot, and hours later I catch them. They always ask, 'Why do you start so slowly?' And I answer, 'Why do you finish so slowly?'"

MOUNTAIN BIKE TERMS

Trail surfaces vary from dirt Forest Service or logging roads to tracks designed and maintained specifically for bikers. Here's an overview:

Singletrack: This is the most common type of trail, approximately the width of one bike; it is ridden single file.

Doubletrack: Typically dirt or gravel backroads that allow bikers to ride side by side.

Bike park: A terrain park that offers a range of downhill and cross-country trails for all skill levels. Visit mtbparks.com to find parks across North America. Many rent equipment.

Flow trail: A long ribbon of roller-coaster-like trail that curves naturally with the landscape or has added features such as bridges, jumps, and banked turns; requires little pedaling or braking as you glide downhill.

Slickrock: Smooth, wind-polished sandstone is a favorite surface of expert bikers.

Gravel: A type of riding that encourages exploration on a variety of surfaces, from gravel to dirt to chert. Use a mapping tool such as Ride with GPS to piece together a custom route. Gravel grinder events welcome everyone from newbies to pros.

Bikes are as varied as the terrain. Here are a few types:

Hardtail: Good for beginners, this all-terrain bike has front suspension and is lighter, easier to maintain, and less expensive.

Fatbike: Wide, oversized tires make this off-road bicycle great for riding on snow, sand, and mud.

E-bike: These hybrid bikes combine traditional pedal power with an electric battery boost.

MOUNTAIN BIKE FUN RIDES

Find a festival or event that matches your skill level on trailforks.com or singletracks.com.

RIDE / LOCATION	TIME

CYCLOCROSS EVENTS

Cyclocross races involve short, timed laps on mostly off-road terrain with obstacles that require riders to carry their bike before continuing on. Prepare to get muddy in a CX race!

RACE	TIME

ROAD BIKING

Lighter frames, thinner tires, longer distances—road biking, or cycling, is more about cardio, the destination, and scenic recreation.

ROAD ROUTES TO TRY

Bike paths, greenways, quiet country roads, and urban avenues are great places to begin. Find local bike trails with AllTrails and TrailLink, and use an app like Strava to track your rides, record your progress, set goals, and connect with local cycling clubs.

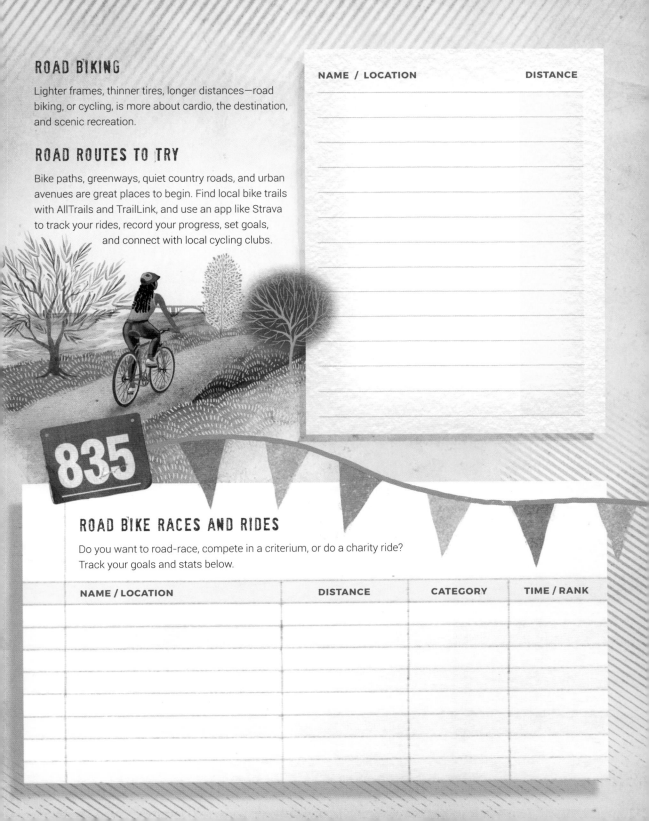

NAME / LOCATION	DISTANCE

835

ROAD BIKE RACES AND RIDES

Do you want to road-race, compete in a criterium, or do a charity ride? Track your goals and stats below.

NAME / LOCATION	DISTANCE	CATEGORY	TIME / RANK

BIKING JOURNAL

Whether off-road or on, use your bike to visit amazing places. Choose six very different locations in your area and cycle there. Take a photo of your bike at each destination, and paste it in below. Do you prefer biking to your favorite outdoor cafe? A secluded beach? A parkway overlook? A mountain pass?

Upload your images to Instagram's #parkedbikesoftheworld, share your experiences, and get inspired by other people's two-wheeled adventures.

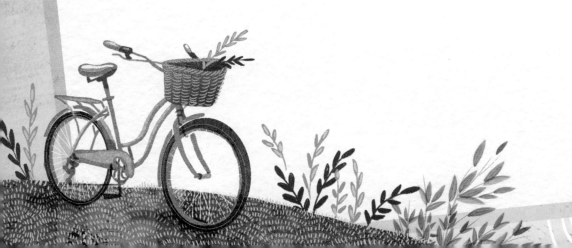

MAP YOUR RIDE!

Commuting by bike is healthy for you and the planet, saves money on gas, and can add a bit of excitement to your daily grind. Mix things up by running errands on your bike or renting a sidewalk bike to check out a fun city destination. Understandably, urban biking can be intimidating because of careless drivers, heavy traffic, and tricky on-the-fly navigation. Make your urban ride smoother and safer by planning your route ahead of time with an app like Strava, Google Maps, or Komoot.

Check out your local cycling club for navigation tips and resources. Some clubs even offer classes to help teach you how to pedal safely around vehicles and pedestrians. After a class or two, you'll feel much more confident on the road.

CLIMB

Rock climbing can be daunting at first. Begin with an introductory class at a local climbing gym, where you can rent a harness and shoes before investing in your own gear. Once you have mastered the basics of tying in to the rope, belaying, and climbing on plastic, you can transition to bouldering and climbing outside, preferably with a mentor. Meetup, Access Fund, Flash Foxy, and Outdoor Women's Alliance are excellent resources for climbing groups in your area—a safe and fun way to get started with experts.

GYM CLIMBING

Gyms provide a safe, controlled climbing experience for all ages and abilities, and are great places to meet new adventure buddies. Most gyms offer a range of classes—everything from technique clinics to yoga—as well as trips to outdoor climbing areas. Get started at a gym near you: climbingbusinessjournal.com/directory/map.

Belaying is the technique of controlling the rope's tension to minimize the distance your partner, the climber, will fall if they slip. When your partner is ready to come down, you (the belayer) take in all the slack and then lower them to the ground.

Auto belays are devices that make it possible to climb on a rope alone in the gym. You simply clip the locking carabiner at the end of the lanyard to your harness (usually the belay loop), lock it, and start climbing. When you weight the lanyard by falling or letting go of the wall, the system will lower you slowly all the way to the ground.

Top roping is the most common style of gym climbing. The climber ties in to one end of a rope that runs up to and through an anchor system. The belayer takes in the rope as the climber ascends.

Lead climbing requires much more skill and knowledge. It involves ascending a route without the protection of a top anchor, while belayed from below. To protect herself should she fall, the climber clips the rope through quickdraws fixed to spaced-out bolts and ultimately, through the anchor at the top. In this scenario, the belayer transitions between feeding out the rope and taking it in.

Footwork is key in climbing. Pull-ups will only get you so far. Instead, focus on your feet. Place them deliberately, then push off smoothly with your legs as you pull down with your arms.

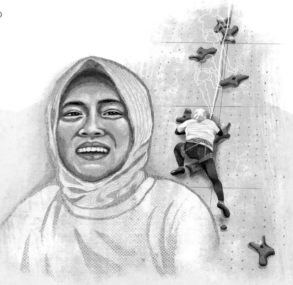

ARIES SUSANTI RAHAYU

"SPIDERWOMAN"

Indonesian speed climber Aries Susanti Rahayu lives up to her superhero nickname. In 2019, she became the first woman to fly up a 15-meter speed wall in less than seven seconds. With the discipline of speed climbing now an Olympic sport, Rahayu is a rising star, not only setting a world record but also shattering barriers for Muslim women—inspiring us all to leap for the impossible.

GYM CLIMBING JOURNAL

What has been the most challenging aspect of indoor climbing for you? How many classes or climbs did it take before you started to feel more confident? Have you taken advantage of all your gym offers—clinics, classes, excursions, film festivals, competitions? Start a list of what you've learned for future reference.

A lot of gym climbers never take the sport outside. If you're interested in checking out your local crag, what might be holding you back? If you prefer to stick to plastic, no pressure! What do you enjoy about climbing indoors?

CLIMBING GRADES Grades are systems for rating the difficulty and skill level of climbs, but they can be somewhat subjective. The Yosemite Decimal System (YDS) applies to routes. Boulder problems are rated on the V-Scale.

Easy: 5.0 to 5.6 — VB
Intermediate to hard: 5.7 to 5.10d — VB to V1
Hard to very difficult: 5.11a to 5.12d — V2 to V6
Extremely difficult: 5.13a to 5.15d — V7 to V16

For 5.10 and above, the grade is typically broken down by letter: 5.10a, 5.10b, 5.10c, 5.10d. Sometimes a plus or minus sign used instead: 5.10− for a 5.10a/b, 5.10+ for a 5.10c/d.

MY STARTING GRADE:

MY CLIMBING GRADE PROGRESS:

BOULDERING

Bouldering is a fun, relatively simple, and economical way to climb. All you need are climbing shoes, a crash pad, chalk, a person to spot you, finger tape, a brush, and a map or guidebook to great boulders. Practice your skills in a gym first, then head out with friends to tackle problems on real rock.

BOULDER PROBLEMS
Keep track of the problems you attempt.

GRADE	NAME / LOCATION

HOW TO FALL WHEN BOULDERING

1. Clear the landing zone of rocks, sticks, and loose gear.

2. Arrange crash pads so they overlap; avoid gaps. Also pad any larger rocks. As you climb, stay over the pads or have your spotter move them as needed.

3. Know where the pad edges are. It can be easy to twist an ankle on the edge of a pad.

4. When you fall or jump off a problem, try to land on your feet with your knees bent. Tuck your head and thumbs in, curl in toward your chest, relax, drop, and roll. Never catch yourself with your hands.

5. Practice these techniques low to the ground until you are comfortable with the skill.

6. Always have at least one trained spotter beneath you. A spotter's job is not to catch you but to help lessen the impact of your fall by guiding your body to the ground safely, with a focus on your torso and head.

SLACKLINING

Walking on a line of webbing similar to a tightrope is the ultimate balancing act. Get started with a beginner ratchet-strap setup: stretch it taut between two trees, about a foot or so off the ground. Balance on one foot, knees slightly bent and your gaze fixed ahead. Practice balancing on the other foot before taking your first steps.

TYPES OF SLACKLINING TO TRY:

WATERLINING is slacklining over water.

RODEOLINING utilizes very loose line tension so that the slackline swings from side to side.

YOGALINING takes traditional yoga poses and moves them onto a slackline.

TRICKLINING uses high tension and stretchy webbing to enable acrobatics like flipping, bouncing, and jumping.

HIGHLINING is slacklining far above the ground. Expert skills, a harness, and a safety leash are a must!

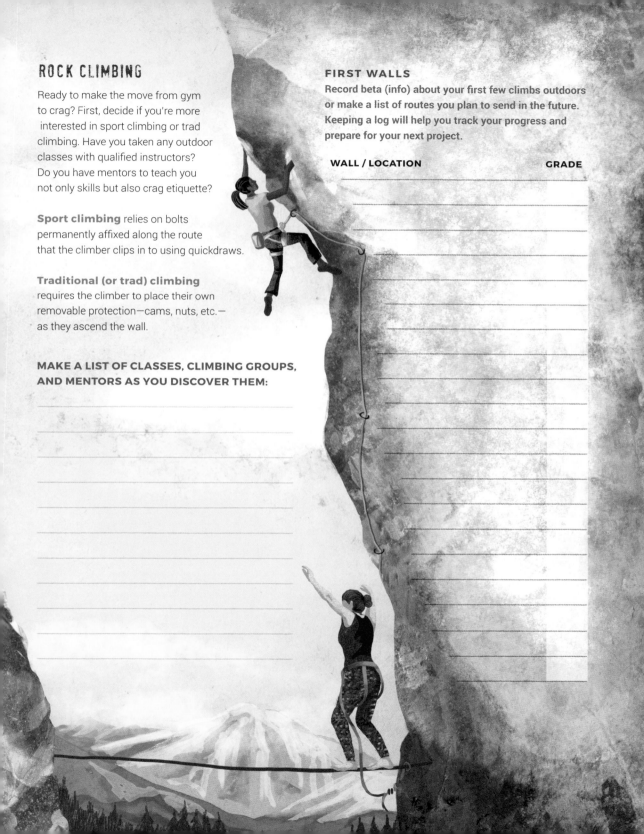

ROCK CLIMBING

Ready to make the move from gym to crag? First, decide if you're more interested in sport climbing or trad climbing. Have you taken any outdoor classes with qualified instructors? Do you have mentors to teach you not only skills but also crag etiquette?

Sport climbing relies on bolts permanently affixed along the route that the climber clips in to using quickdraws.

Traditional (or trad) climbing requires the climber to place their own removable protection—cams, nuts, etc.— as they ascend the wall.

MAKE A LIST OF CLASSES, CLIMBING GROUPS, AND MENTORS AS YOU DISCOVER THEM:

FIRST WALLS

Record beta (info) about your first few climbs outdoors or make a list of routes you plan to send in the future. Keeping a log will help you track your progress and prepare for your next project.

WALL / LOCATION	GRADE

JUNKO TABEI

PIONEERING MOUNTAINEER

Japanese mountaineer Junko Tabei was the first woman to summit Mount Everest, reaching the world's highest point in 1975. Breaking down even more barriers, Tabei also became the first woman to climb the Seven Summits, the highest peak on each continent. She continued climbing well into her later years, living to the age of seventy-seven.

"Anyone with a pair of feet who can walk can climb," she said. "The most important thing is not being concerned about having the money, time, or skills to climb, but the desire. Don't think too hard. Just do it."

"I'm a free spirit. Call me the free spirit of the mountains."

OUTDOOR CLIMBING JOURNAL

Fear is a good thing—it is our body's natural response to danger, designed to keep us safe. However, successful climbers learn to manage *perceived* "dangers," such as the fear of taking a safe lead fall, versus *real* dangers like loose rock or a dicey runout. Be realistic about your personal ability, training, experience, gear, and safety backups. Only climb routes you feel prepared to tackle.

What mental techniques help bring you back from fear—focusing on your breath, visualizing the moves ahead, or perhaps reciting a mantra? How did you feel when you first succeeded on a route—elation, relief, a mix of the two? Think about how far you want to take the sport: Do you want to climb higher grades, visit destination areas, or just have fun at the crag on the weekend with friends?

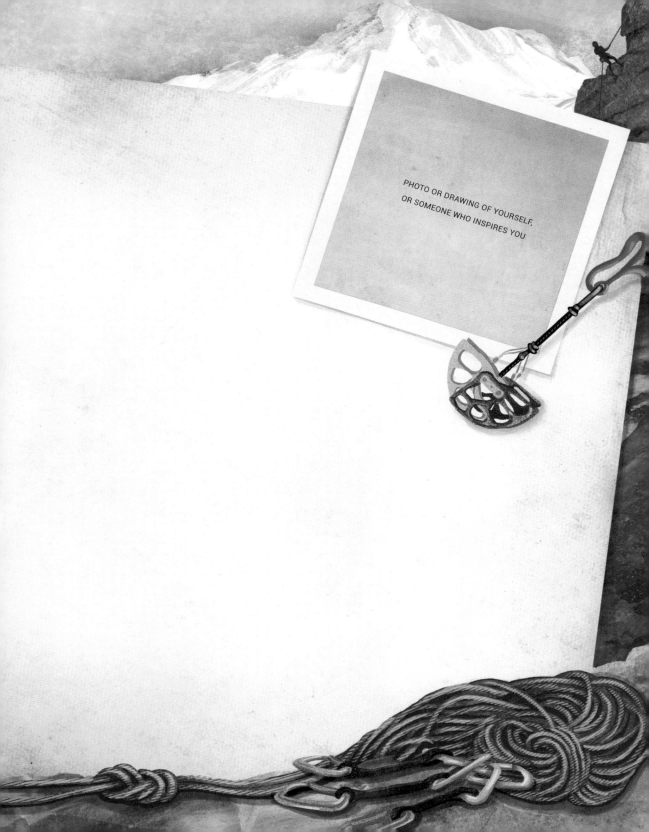

PHOTO OR DRAWING OF YOURSELF,
OR SOMEONE WHO INSPIRES YOU

THE SEVEN SUMMITS

ACONCAGUA
SOUTH AMERICA
22,841 FT / 6962 M

MOUNT KILIMANJARO
AFRICA
19,340 FT / 5895 M

VINSON MASSIF
ANTARCTICA
16,050 FT / 4892 M

MOUNT EVEREST
ASIA
29,035 FT / 8850 M

EVEREST BASE CAMP
17,600 FT / 5364 M

DENALI
NORTH AMERICA
20,320 FT / 6194 M

MOUNT ELBRUS
EUROPE
18,510 FT / 5642 M

PUNCAK JAYA
CARSTENZ PYRAMID; OCEANIA
16,023 FT / 4884 M

Do you aspire to tackle one of the world's tallest peaks? It's possible to achieve your dream with careful planning, diligent training, the right gear, and a fee for an outfitter and permit. Trekking companies offer many options to get you to one or more of the Seven Summits, the highest peak on each continent. Some of these mountains require little technical mountaineering experience, while others demand a high level of skill.

A determined, positive outlook and a drive to succeed are crucial. (Even if Everest is out of reach, a trek to Everest Base Camp to see the Khumbu Icefall is a worthy, less pricey goal.)

Days before we summited Kilimanjaro, my guide Nick Basso said, "Kilimanjaro is challenging. You meet yourself on the mountain." Do you want to see what you're made of?

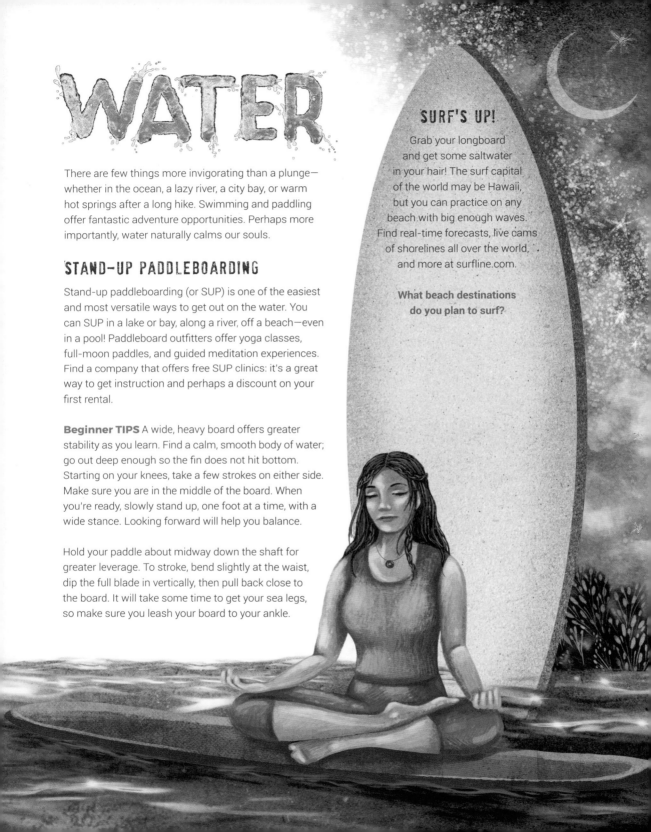

WATER

There are few things more invigorating than a plunge—whether in the ocean, a lazy river, a city bay, or warm hot springs after a long hike. Swimming and paddling offer fantastic adventure opportunities. Perhaps more importantly, water naturally calms our souls.

STAND-UP PADDLEBOARDING

Stand-up paddleboarding (or SUP) is one of the easiest and most versatile ways to get out on the water. You can SUP in a lake or bay, along a river, off a beach—even in a pool! Paddleboard outfitters offer yoga classes, full-moon paddles, and guided meditation experiences. Find a company that offers free SUP clinics: it's a great way to get instruction and perhaps a discount on your first rental.

Beginner TIPS A wide, heavy board offers greater stability as you learn. Find a calm, smooth body of water; go out deep enough so the fin does not hit bottom. Starting on your knees, take a few strokes on either side. Make sure you are in the middle of the board. When you're ready, slowly stand up, one foot at a time, with a wide stance. Looking forward will help you balance.

Hold your paddle about midway down the shaft for greater leverage. To stroke, bend slightly at the waist, dip the full blade in vertically, then pull back close to the board. It will take some time to get your sea legs, so make sure you leash your board to your ankle.

SURF'S UP!

Grab your longboard and get some saltwater in your hair! The surf capital of the world may be Hawaii, but you can practice on any beach with big enough waves. Find real-time forecasts, live cams of shorelines all over the world, and more at surfline.com.

What beach destinations do you plan to surf?

WATER NOTES

At the beginning of my career, I sat under the fluorescent lights of my Washington, DC, office longing to be standing barefoot in water under a canopy of trees. Splashing in my local creek was a highlight of my childhood, and it remains a sacred place. Now my favorite summertime treat is to swim at midnight under a full moon with friends. What is your relationship to water? Do you find it soul-cleansing, or do its dark depths scare you a bit? Are you brave enough to try an icy polar bear plunge or deep-sea scuba diving? What is your most memorable—terrifying, rejuvenating, exhilarating—experience of being in or on the water?

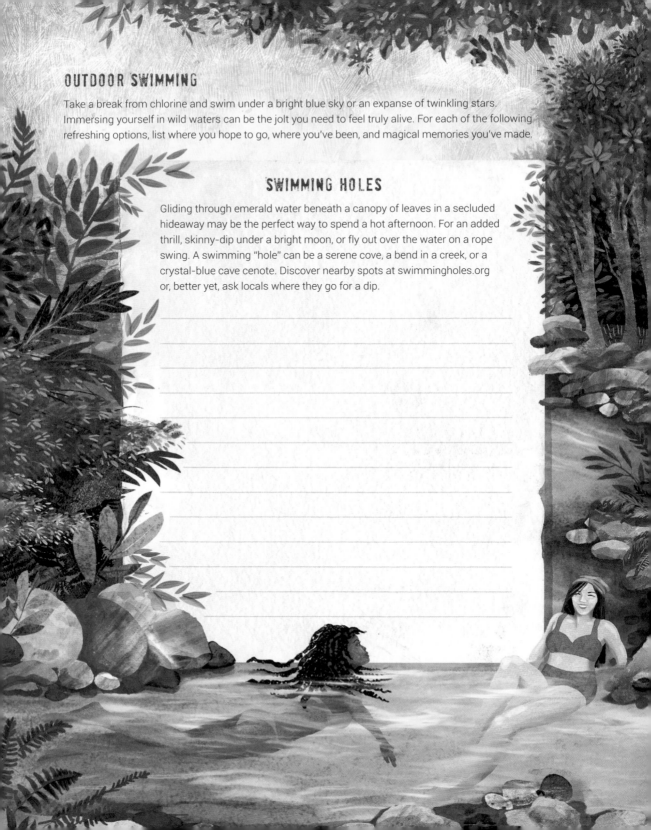

OUTDOOR SWIMMING

Take a break from chlorine and swim under a bright blue sky or an expanse of twinkling stars. Immersing yourself in wild waters can be the jolt you need to feel truly alive. For each of the following refreshing options, list where you hope to go, where you've been, and magical memories you've made.

SWIMMING HOLES

Gliding through emerald water beneath a canopy of leaves in a secluded hideaway may be the perfect way to spend a hot afternoon. For an added thrill, skinny-dip under a bright moon, or fly out over the water on a rope swing. A swimming "hole" can be a serene cove, a bend in a creek, or a crystal-blue cave cenote. Discover nearby spots at swimmingholes.org or, better yet, ask locals where they go for a dip.

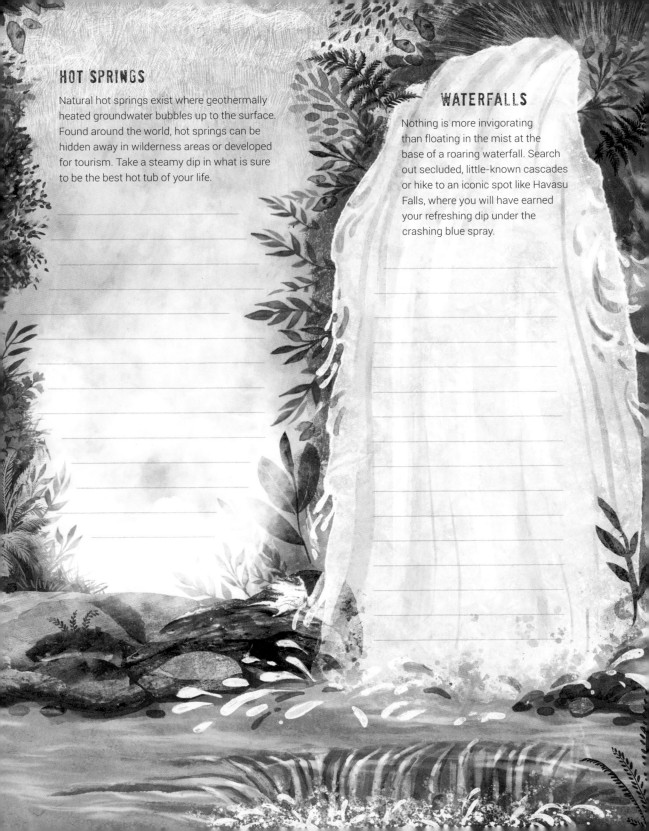

HOT SPRINGS

Natural hot springs exist where geothermally heated groundwater bubbles up to the surface. Found around the world, hot springs can be hidden away in wilderness areas or developed for tourism. Take a steamy dip in what is sure to be the best hot tub of your life.

WATERFALLS

Nothing is more invigorating than floating in the mist at the base of a roaring waterfall. Search out secluded, little-known cascades or hike to an iconic spot like Havasu Falls, where you will have earned your refreshing dip under the crashing blue spray.

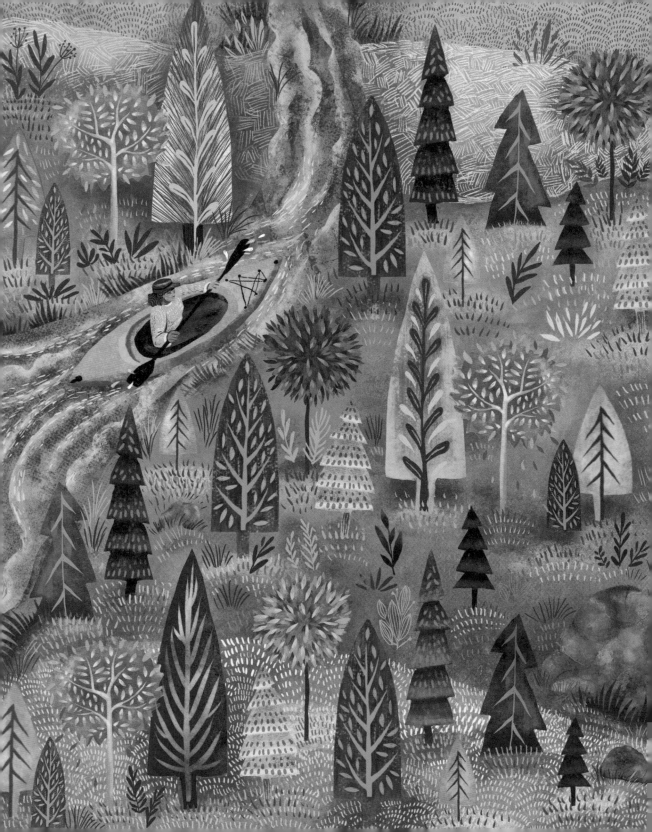

CANOEING AND KAYAKING

I introduced my toddler son to kayaking by tucking him in front of me in his tiny life jacket with a bag of snacks. He was never calmer than on those balmy days spent gliding down the Piney River. When he was a teenager, we embarked on a four-day, 101-mile river paddle, camping in a hammock along its banks. Adventures are far more than bucket list items; they allow you to create lifelong bonds with the people you love.

KNOW YOUR BOATS

When selecting a boat, think about your intended use and the type of water you'll be on. Do you plan to paddle across a placid lake, navigate some rapids, or head to sea?

Classic canoes are ideal for a two-person adventure—or an outing with young children—on quiet water like a lake, slow river, or protected bay.

Recreational kayaks are popular with beginners. They are heavy, usually made of hard plastic, and quite stable on flat water, small inland lakes, and slow rivers. Their wide, sit-in cockpits make getting in and out of the boat easy. They are *not* appropriate for large, choppy bodies of water that could easily swamp the hull and sink the boat.

Sit-on-top kayaks are also made of plastic, open on top, and perfect for general recreational use in warmer weather, sort of like a giant raft. These boats have self-draining holes; if a sit-on-top flips, you can turn it upright and hop back on.

Crossover kayaks are great for touring both calm and choppier water. The rounded bow helps keep the water below you.

Touring kayaks are long, narrow boats intended for speed and comfort over long-distance paddles.

Sea kayaks are often made of fiberglass, making them lightweight, and they have sealed bulkheads at the bow and stern filled with air. Should the boat flip, the bulkheads will keep it afloat. They are designed for paddling in the ocean or other open, unpredictable water. A spray skirt can keep you dry and prevent water from filling the hull.

Whitewater kayaks have smaller cockpits with fitted spray skirts. They are shorter with a rounded design for greater maneuverability in rapids.

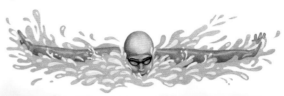

YUSRA MARDINI

SYRIAN REFUGEE AND OLYMPIC SWIMMER

Fleeing civil war in Syria, Yusra Mardini and her sister Sara attempted a sea crossing from Turkey to Greece in a dinghy full of fellow refugees. Within fifteen minutes the boat engine had failed and twenty people were at risk of drowning. Mardini, Sara, and two others jumped overboard and towed the dinghy for more than three hours, saving everyone. A year later, Mardini joined the first-ever Refugee Olympic Team and competed in swimming at the 2016 Rio Olympics. She continues her work as a goodwill ambassador and is training for the postponed Tokyo Olympics.

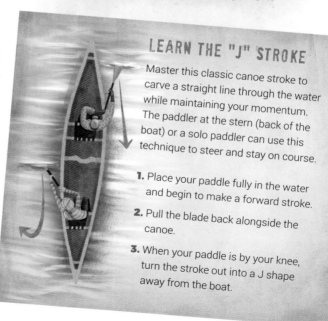

LEARN THE "J" STROKE

Master this classic canoe stroke to carve a straight line through the water while maintaining your momentum. The paddler at the stern (back of the boat) or a solo paddler can use this technique to steer and stay on course.

1. Place your paddle fully in the water and begin to make a forward stroke.

2. Pull the blade back alongside the canoe.

3. When your paddle is by your knee, turn the stroke out into a J shape away from the boat.

WHITEWATER RAFTING

Imagine plunging down rapids surrounded by towering canyon walls or taking an exhilarating ride through a forested valley on a wild-and-scenic river. While whitewater kayaking is strictly for expert-level paddlers, whitewater *rafting* is much more accessible, with guided trips available across the US for everyone from beginners to experienced thrill-seekers. Meander through gentle rapids with the whole family on a half-day trip. Feed your adrenaline-junkie side with a more rough-and-tumble multiday outing. Although many popular rafting rivers are located in the West, the world's largest paddling festival takes place every September on the Gauley River in West Virginia. For a unique rafting experience, consider running the 1996 Olympics course on the Ocoee River in Tennessee.

ADD A PHOTO OF YOUR CREW!

RAPID CLASSIFICATIONS

Class I: Relaxing, small waves; great for beginners

Class II: Easy waves with some rocks or small drops

Class III: Medium waves, drops, and a fast current that requires experienced paddling

Class IV: Difficult, turbulent whitewater; demands precise, advanced maneuvering

Class V: Complex, large, continuous rapids with big drops and large rocks; expert skills required

Record the details of your first few river trips:

RIVER NAME / LOCATION / OUTFITTER	RAPIDS CLASSIFICATION

PADDLING JOURNAL

What kind of paddling did you try? Do you prefer gliding across a smooth lake or navigating rapids on a multiday expedition? Use this space to reflect on your paddling experiences or to brainstorm a big whitewater or canoe-camping adventure.

SNOW

Crystal-clear nights, tree branches heavy with fresh powder, crack-ling fires to warm your bones—I crave winter's cozy quiet. It's a time to hibernate, go inward, and dream up plans, trips, and projects for the coming year. The short, crisp, chilly days can be energizing as well. After the season's first snowfall, I drop everything and head to the woods for a long hike in the newly hushed forest.

Grab a mug of your favorite hot drink and think about what makes the season magical to you. Do you love carving down ski slopes through fresh powder, ice skating with friends, or listening to the crunch of snow beneath your boots on a long solo walk? Or do you find yourself yearning for the sunny days of summer? If so, what aspects of winter can you try to embrace? Fill this space with plans for the season.

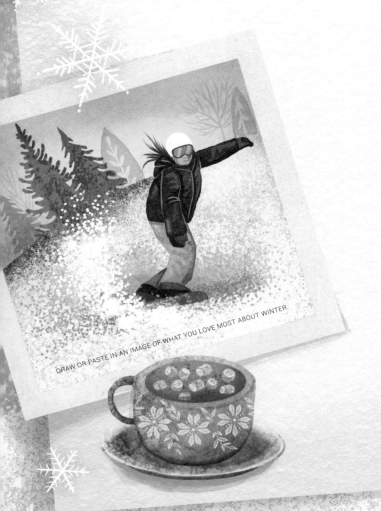

DRAW OR PASTE IN AN IMAGE OF WHAT YOU LOVE MOST ABOUT WINTER

BARBARA HILLARY

POLAR ADVENTURER

Proving that you are never too old to pursue your dreams, Barbara Hillary made history at the age of seventy-five by becoming the first-known African American woman to stand on the North Pole. Less than four years later, Hillary broke the same barrier at the South Pole.

"Negative people told me, 'You're too old. As a lung cancer survivor, your lungs will never be able to tolerate the incredible cold weather,'" she said. Rising out of childhood poverty and surviving two different kinds of cancer, Hillary was determined to keep life interesting, even after her retirement. "It's a matter of believing in yourself. And if I failed, so what—I tried." But succeed she did, reaching the top (and bottom) of the world!

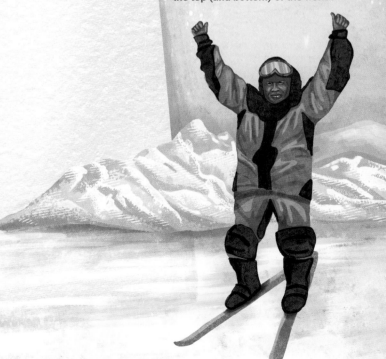

SNOWBOARDING

Start out practicing these board tricks on flat terrain. Beginners should seek out soft, fresh snow; it can be very difficult to stop or control your speed on icy or hardpacked snow.

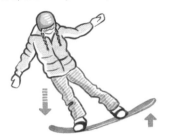

TAIL PRESS

Get your hips over the tail of your board and bend your back knee until the nose of the board flexes off the ground.

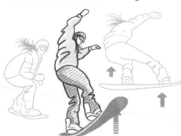

OLLIE

Originally a skateboard trick, the ollie involves leaning back with your hips over the tail of your board until it flexes. Use the energy of the flex to pop your board into the air. Pull your legs into your chest to get even more height.

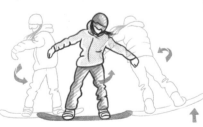

BUTTER SPIN

Wind your body and jump up to spin the board while leaning into a tail press.

DOWNHILL SKIING

Also known as alpine skiing, this winter sport allows you to glide down slopes on skis with fixed-heel bindings that help you control your turns and speed.

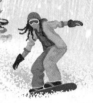
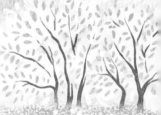

SKI AND SNOWBOARD RENTAL TIPS

Here's some general advice to get a good fit when you are renting gear at a ski resort.

Helmet: Your helmet should fit snugly but not be too tight. Shake your head up and down and from side to side. If the helmet moves or shifts, size down. Make sure it works well with your goggles and does not hinder your vision.

Skis: Shorter, softer, narrower skis are the best bet for beginners. Choose a pair that reaches between your nose and eyebrows when you stand them upright.

Snowboard: If you are just starting out, select an all-mountain or freestyle board that has soft to medium flex. Standing on one end, the board should hit between your nose and chin.

Boots: Wear a single pair of thin, wool or synthetic ski or snowboard socks. A soft-flex boot is great for beginners. Take out the liner, and place your foot in the shell; you want roughly two fingers' width behind your heel. Put the liner back into the boot and make sure your feet fit snugly but don't feel cramped. There should be no pressure points.

Poles: While standing in your boots, turn a pole upside down, grip it underneath the basket, and check that your arm bends at a ninety-degree angle when the top of the pole rests on the ground.

You'll also want to get a pair of goggles to protect your eyes and appropriate clothing to keep you warm. Dress in layers, and don't forget socks and gloves or mittens.

HIT THE SLOPES!

Not everyone lives within easy
driving distance of ski slopes. If you
already alpine ski or snowboard, list
the resorts and areas you hope to
visit. If you've never strapped on a
snowboard or alpine skis and want
to try, research nearby ski areas
and the classes they offer, then
make a plan to start below.

RESORT / LOCATION

_____

_____

_____

_____

_____

_____

_____

_____

_____

_____

_____

CLASS NOTES

Ski resorts offer instruction for skiers and
boarders of all skill levels. Note the tips, tricks,
and techniques you learn in class and practice
until you level up!

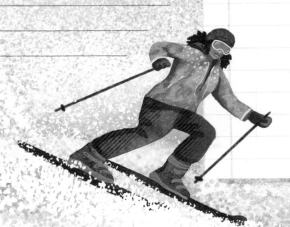

SNOWSHOEING

Strap a pair of snowshoes over your warm waterproof boots and take a hike! Trekking poles with snow baskets will make your walk easier. Many resorts have wooded trails to explore—a great option if ski conditions up high aren't perfect. Be sure to wear ski or rain pants with a base layer to stay dry.

Layering is important for both snowshoeing and cross-country skiing. It's best to start out chilly because you'll soon warm up from exertion. Always carry the Ten Essentials in a day pack. Treat yourself by adding a thermos of your favorite warm drink.

If you'll be snowshoeing in the backcountry, take classes about avalanche preparedness and pack the necessary safety equipment. With the sport's growing popularity, some competitions such as winter quadrathlons have added a snowshoe component.

CROSS-COUNTRY SKIING

Glide over beautiful, snowy terrain for an aerobic work-out or meander along groomed trails while admiring the winter wonderland around you. Also known as Nordic skiing, cross-country (XC) skiing features a free-heel binding system: your toe clicks in to the binding while your heel remains unattached and free to maneuver. The easiest style to begin with is classic skiing. Simply step into the groomed tracks and stride forward on one ski, then the other, while pushing with the opposite pole—similar to the natural rhythm of walking.

The other popular style is skate skiing, which resembles speed skating in that you push off in diagonal strides to propel yourself forward. Skate skiing works best on hard, compact snow and requires wide, groomed trails.

Find trails and classes for beginners at resorts across the US and Canada at xcski.org. If racing piques your interest, consider entering the Yellowstone Rendezvous Race, with 10K, 25K, and 50K options. What a great way to see a national park!

ANATOMY OF A SNOWSHOE

Historians believe snowshoes were used in central Asia as far back as 6000 years ago. When the ancestors of Native Americans and the Inuit migrated into North America, they brought early versions of wooden and rawhide snowshoes. Modern snowshoes use the same principles, but the materials have evolved to make a day of trekking easy for all ages and fitness levels.

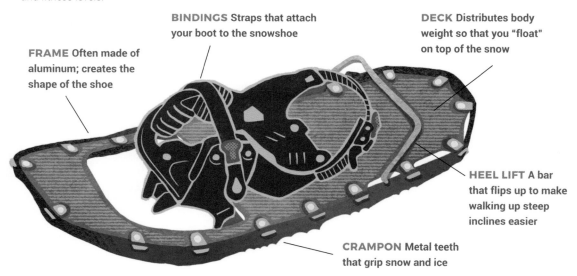

BINDINGS Straps that attach your boot to the snowshoe

DECK Distributes body weight so that you "float" on top of the snow

FRAME Often made of aluminum; creates the shape of the shoe

HEEL LIFT A bar that flips up to make walking up steep inclines easier

CRAMPON Metal teeth that grip snow and ice

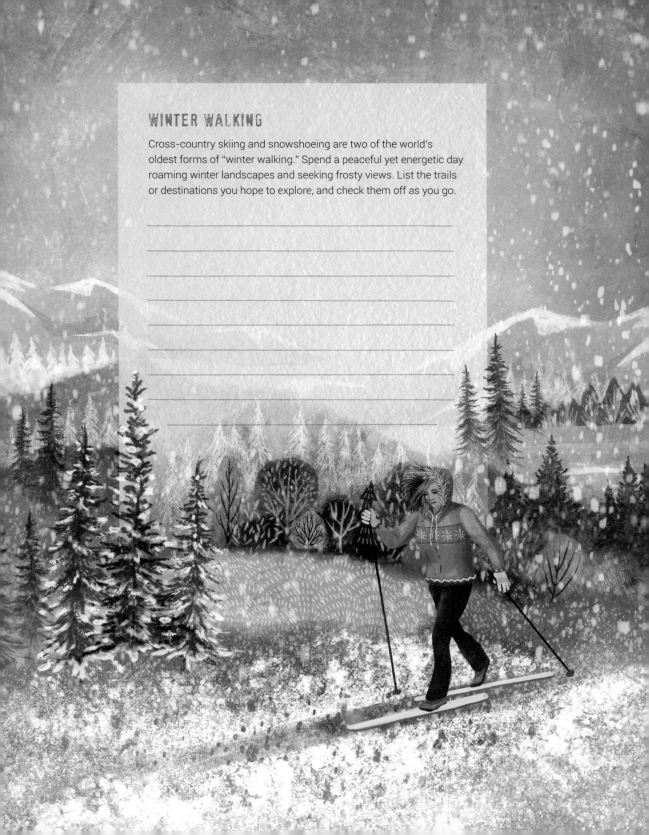

WINTER WALKING

Cross-country skiing and snowshoeing are two of the world's oldest forms of "winter walking." Spend a peaceful yet energetic day roaming winter landscapes and seeking frosty views. List the trails or destinations you hope to explore, and check them off as you go.

_____

_____

_____

_____

_____

_____

_____

_____

SKI BIKING

Blast downhill at parks and resorts on what is essentially a bike frame mounted on skis.

A FEW WELL-KNOWN DESTINATIONS:
Aspen, Colorado
Breckenridge, Colorado
Durango, Colorado
Brighton, Utah
Pats Peak, New Hampshire
Sun Peaks, BC, Canada

PARK OR RESORT / LOCATION

_____

_____

_____

_____

For cross-country riding in winter, try fatbiking, where wider tires offer improved grip and stability on snowy trails and forest roads.

The Iditarod Trail Invitational is an ultramarathon that takes its hardy participants 350 or 1000 miles across Alaskan wilderness in brutal winter conditions—on bike, foot, or skis.

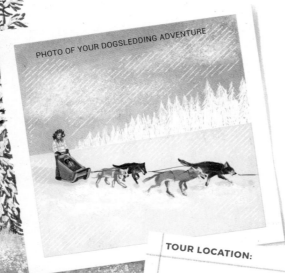

PHOTO OF YOUR DOGSLEDDING ADVENTURE

TOUR LOCATION:

ICE SKATING

A winter classic! Glide across a frozen pond or practice your spins at a local rink, which typically offer rentals. You can also search for used ice skates on Craigslist or at Goodwill shops. If you venture out to a local lake or pond, make sure the temps have been below freezing for at least a week and confirm that the ice is four inches thick at minimum. In some northern states and provinces, "wild skating"—skating on a remote mountain lake or along a frozen river—has become popular. In these harsher environments, be prepared for rough and rippled surfaces and wear a pair of ice claws around your neck for safety.

Describe your first skating experience:

DOGSLEDDING

Enjoy this winter activity that originated thousands of years ago as a means of transportation for Inuit and other northern Native peoples. As snowmobiles began to replace dog teams in the 1950s, Alaska's famed Iditarod Trail Sled Dog Race was created to preserve traditional sled dog culture. Today, many ski resorts and outfitters in snow-rich regions—New England, the Great Lakes, the West, and Alaska—offer dogsled excursions to icefields, glaciers, and other backcountry destinations. For a unique winter sport, try skijoring—cross-country skiing while pulled by a dog or horse. A warm-weather alternative: skatejoring with rollerblades or a skateboard.

LEARN SOME BASIC SLED COMMANDS:
Gee! Turn right.   **Hike!** or **Let's Go!** Start moving.
Haw! Turn left.   **Whoa!** Stop.

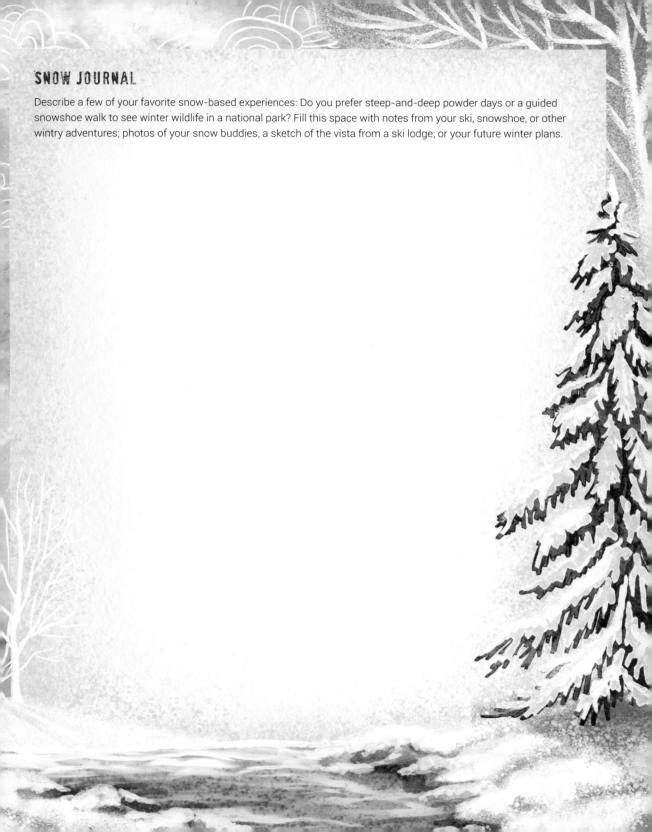

SNOW JOURNAL

Describe a few of your favorite snow-based experiences: Do you prefer steep-and-deep powder days or a guided snowshoe walk to see winter wildlife in a national park? Fill this space with notes from your ski, snowshoe, or other wintry adventures; photos of your snow buddies; a sketch of the vista from a ski lodge; or your future winter plans.

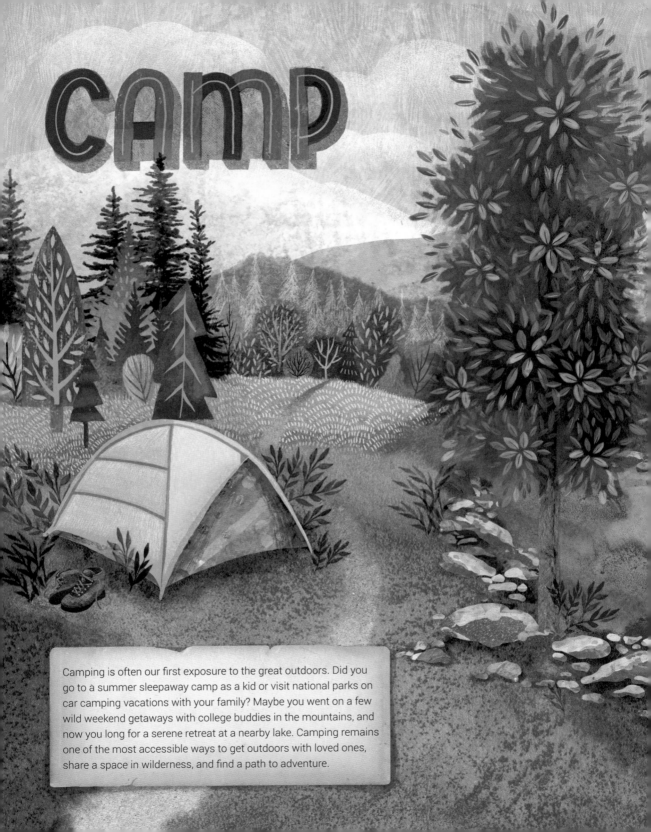

CAMP

Camping is often our first exposure to the great outdoors. Did you go to a summer sleepaway camp as a kid or visit national parks on car camping vacations with your family? Maybe you went on a few wild weekend getaways with college buddies in the mountains, and now you long for a serene retreat at a nearby lake. Camping remains one of the most accessible ways to get outdoors with loved ones, share a space in wilderness, and find a path to adventure.

CAR CAMPING

WHAT I PACK

Below is my checklist of must-have items for car camping. I tailor it to suit the location, weather forecast, and planned activities.

Shelter: Tent, footprint, hammock

Sleep system: Sleeping bag in a compression sack, liner, pad, inflatable pillow

Chair: A compact backpacking-style one

Food: Meals, coffee, snacks

Cooking and campfire-related gear: Stove, fuel, lighter, knife, tinder, thin cutting board, pot, cup, bowl, utensils, French press, camp soap, sponge, paper towels, trash bags

Hydration: Bottled drinking water, water bottles, and a filtration system

Clothing: Socks, underwear, sports bra, pants, shirts, leggings, base layer for sleeping, warm jacket, hat, raingear, boots, camp shoes

Bathroom: Toilet paper, trowel, hand sanitizer, baby wipes, sealable plastic bags to pack out trash

Toiletries: Toothbrush and paste, contacts and glasses, comb, mirror, hair ties, prescription medications, camp towel

The Ten Essentials: See list in "Backpacking," plus insect repellent

Extra gear: Day pack, inflatable solar lantern, nylon cord, hiking poles, carabiners

Communication: Cell phone, charging block

Luxury items: Travel watercolor kit, book, oracle cards, and incense!

YOUR CAR CAMPING CHECKLIST

Make your own checklist and keep a copy with your gear so you can consult it as you pack for each trip.

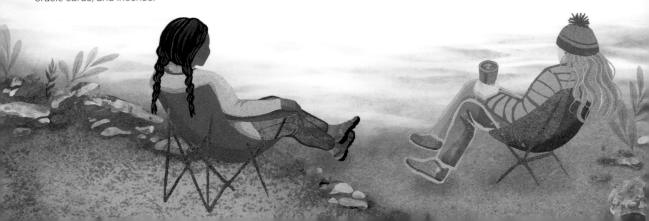

CAMPGROUND SKILLS

Camping requires some important but easy-to-learn skills: planning and organizing a trip, setting up a tent, tying knots, preparing food, purifying water, and filleting a trout, to name a few. But the most essential may be building a campfire. Be responsible and follow the Leave No Trace principles described earlier in the hiking section for a safe and fun campfire experience! Always fully extinguish your campfire before you leave or go to sleep.

To start a fire, you'll need some highly combustible material known as tinder. Bring one or two options on your camping trips:

- **Fatwood:** Purchase a small bundle of these 100 percent natural heartwood pine sticks from any home improvement or outdoor store. Each piece is concentrated with resin and will light quickly, even if damp. Shave off pieces with a knife or light the whole stick.

- **Wood shavings:** Use your knife to whittle a few dry sticks.

- **Natural materials:** Collect pine needles, dry dead leaves, or fine, bark-like birch.

- **Vaseline-coated cotton balls:** Dip the cotton in petroleum jelly and store in a plastic bag. Pull the cotton apart before lighting.

- **Cotton tampon:** Remove all packaging and fluff it out or tear it into pieces.

- **Tea bags:** Dry out your used tea bags and coat them in leftover candle wax.

HOW TO START A FIRE

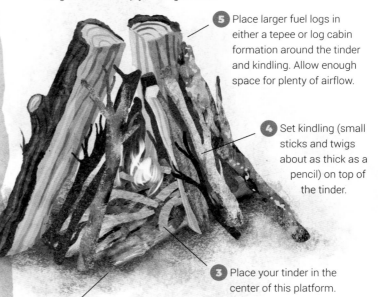

1 Place all the materials you will need near an existing fire pit: bark or sticks, tinder, kindling, larger logs, and a lighter, preferably one with a long handle to keep your fingers safe.

5 Place larger fuel logs in either a tepee or log cabin formation around the tinder and kindling. Allow enough space for plenty of airflow.

4 Set kindling (small sticks and twigs about as thick as a pencil) on top of the tinder.

3 Place your tinder in the center of this platform.

2 First lay the bark or sticks on the bottom of the pit to create a dry platform.

6 Light the tinder. Blowing from the side may help ignite the sparks.

7 Once the kindling is burning, gradually add larger pieces of wood as needed.

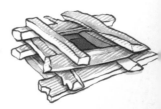

Tepee
Arrange sticks into a cone shape, leaning against each other.

Log Cabin
Stack pieces of wood two at a time on opposite sides. Alternate pairs to form a box shape.

CAMP STOVES & TOOLS

The other critical part of successful car camping? Good food! It's easy enough to cook over an open fire pit, but bringing a camp stove allows you to prepare gourmet meals.

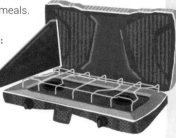

Propane camp stove: Great for beginners, this two-burner stove runs on propane. You can adjust the heat to simmer, sauté, and boil as needed.

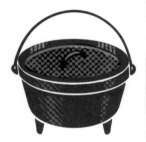

Butane single-burner stove: A smaller, more compact portable stove may be all you need. Cook in a single pot or pan.

Dutch oven: While Dutch ovens are heavy, they are perhaps the most versatile option. Make a stew, cook lasagna, and bake cookies or a cobbler—all in a single pot over hot coals.

Camp grill: Use a foldable, lightweight grill to cook burgers, kebabs, hot dogs— you name it!—over campfire coals.

Wood-burning camp stove: This stove runs by burning sticks, twigs, or pine cones inside its chamber. Turn fire into electricity and charge your devices via a built-in USB port while cooking dinner! It is versatile—able to handle heavy cookware and yet suitable for backpacking.

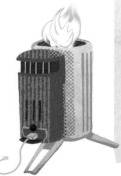

CAMPFIRE FUN

A roaring campfire is the perfect setting for guitar playing, storytelling, sing-alongs, and word games. I love sharing my real paranormal experiences from when I lived in a haunted house. Do you have a classic ghost tale that will keep everyone awake at night?

Make a list of your favorite songs, games, and tall tales.

Spend the night at a legendary haunted campground—if you dare! Here are a few to get you started:

**Antietam Creek Campsite, Maryland
Big Moose Lake, New York
Holy Ghost Campground, New Mexico
Lake Morena, California
Montgomery Bell State Park, Tennessee
Vallecito Stage Station County Park
Campground, California**

CAMP COOKING

What is your favorite easy meal to make at camp? Keep a small notebook of cooking ideas with your camping gear for quick reference when you're planning your next trip. Here's my favorite go-to camping meal.

BUILD YOUR OWN FOIL-PACK DINNER

There is nothing better when camping than a foil-pack dinner. Each person can get creative and experiment with spices and toppings to build their custom meal. Feeding vegetarians, meat lovers, or picky eaters? No problem.

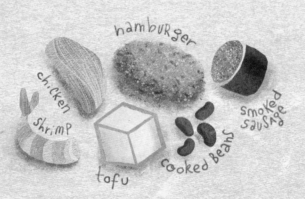

1 Bring a selection of precut proteins.

TIP Freeze meat before packing. It will last longer in your cooler as it safely thaws.

2 Prepare a variety of colorful veggies. Cut potatoes and carrots small or thin so they will cook in the same amount of time as softer vegetables.

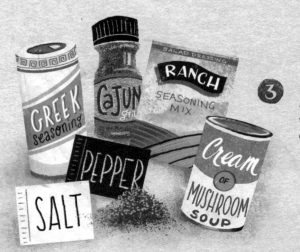

3 Pack a variety of dried herbs and spices. A tablespoon or two of canned soup makes a creamy gravy.

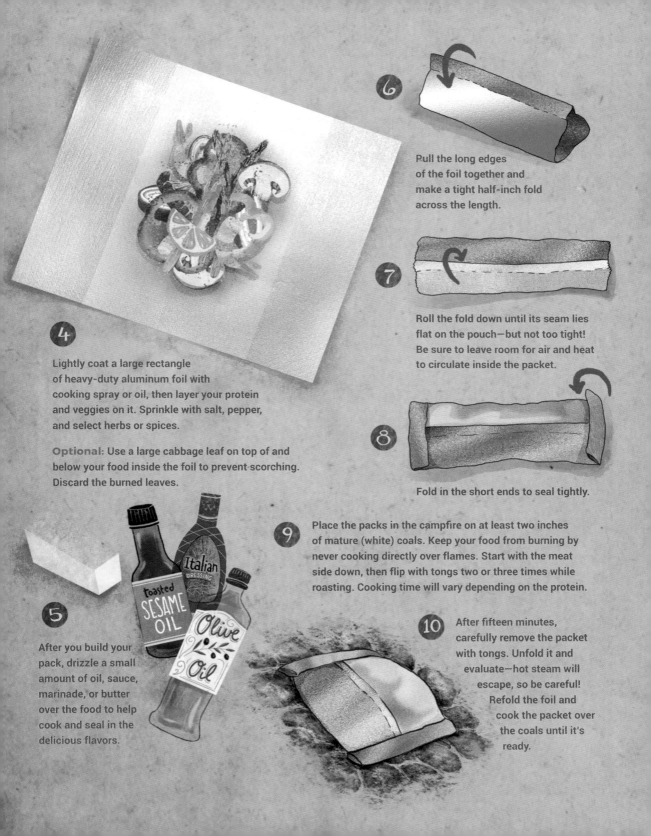

6

Pull the long edges of the foil together and make a tight half-inch fold across the length.

7

Roll the fold down until its seam lies flat on the pouch—but not too tight! Be sure to leave room for air and heat to circulate inside the packet.

8

Fold in the short ends to seal tightly.

4

Lightly coat a large rectangle of heavy-duty aluminum foil with cooking spray or oil, then layer your protein and veggies on it. Sprinkle with salt, pepper, and select herbs or spices.

Optional: Use a large cabbage leaf on top of and below your food inside the foil to prevent scorching. Discard the burned leaves.

5

After you build your pack, drizzle a small amount of oil, sauce, marinade, or butter over the food to help cook and seal in the delicious flavors.

9

Place the packs in the campfire on at least two inches of mature (white) coals. Keep your food from burning by never cooking directly over flames. Start with the meat side down, then flip with tongs two or three times while roasting. Cooking time will vary depending on the protein.

10

After fifteen minutes, carefully remove the packet with tongs. Unfold it and evaluate—hot steam will escape, so be careful! Refold the foil and cook the packet over the coals until it's ready.

fall asleep under the stars

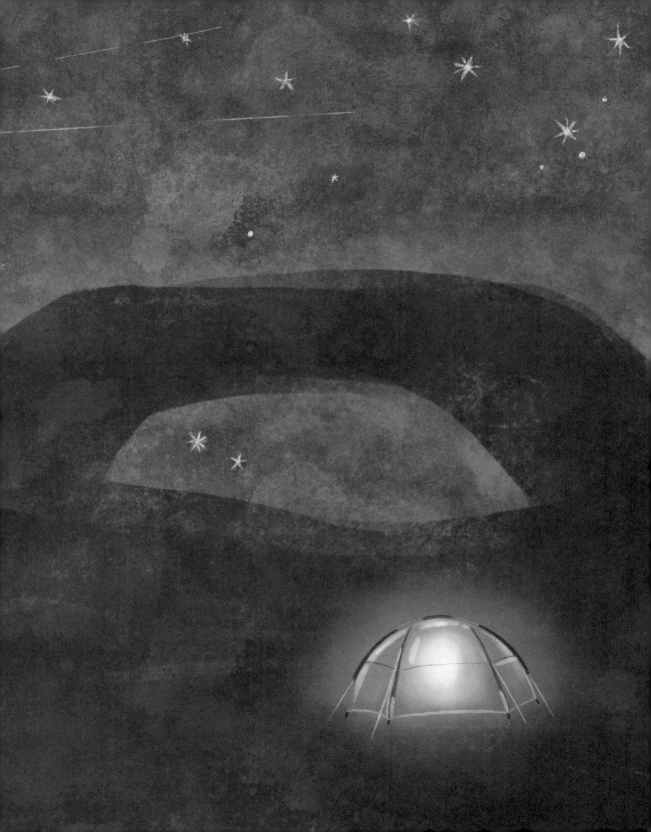

SHELTER

A safe space that shields us from the elements—it is a basic human need. With camping shelters ranging from glamorous to bare minimum, there is no "one right way" to sleep outside. Find what works for you and enjoy a night under the stars!

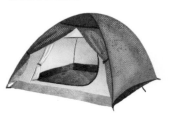

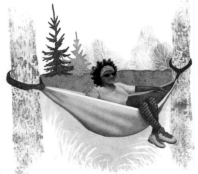

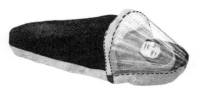

Tent: There are numerous styles to choose from. Whether you go with a multiroom setup or an ultralight, one-person backpacking design, tents offer great protection from rain, snow, wind, and bugs. Three-season tents tend to be lighter and more breathable. Four-season tents can handle winter weather and more extreme conditions.

Hammock: If you hate sleeping on the ground and it's not too cold, a hammock may be the answer! They are super lightweight and simple to set up. You may want to add a tarp or mosquito netting.

Bivy sack: Are you a minimalist? A bivy sack is an ultralight slipcover that fits over your pad and sleeping bag. Originally used as emergency protection for climbers, a bivy is the perfect grab-and-go option for a spontaneous night outside when the forecast is good.

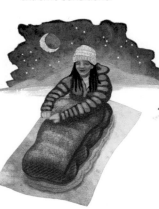

Cowboy camping: It's like in the old westerns—just you in your sleeping bag, out in the open. Talk about freedom!

Trail shelters: These three-sided, Adirondack lean-to log structures with a platform can be found in parks across America and along the Appalachian Trail. Sleeping in one is like spending the night in an open-air cabin.

Glamping: Take your car camping to the next level with some glamour! String up solar-powered party lights, unpack your fancy wine glasses, and serve chocolate-dipped strawberries. Fill your hammock with fringed pillows and colorful quilts. Glamping campgrounds offer yurts or large canvas tents with beds and furniture. It's about being over the top and having fun!

TIP Peruse Hipcamp to book unusual camping experiences like hammock-glamping in a cabana or pitching your tent at a farm sanctuary.

SLEEPING WARM

When sleeping, women tend to have much lower internal body temperatures than men. Our blood supply gets pulled from our extremities toward our core and reproductive organs, leaving us with chilly feet and hands. Women's-specific sleeping bags are designed with this in mind, though temperature rating and fit should be your most important considerations when shopping for a bag.

Here are a few tips for staying cozy while you snooze:

Sleep in a hat. If you forgot to pack one, transform a T-shirt into a makeshift beanie.

Set aside a pair of sleep socks. Keep a pair of wool or fleece socks in your bag reserved for sleeping.

Change your clothes! Start the night in dry clothes.

Sleep on an insulated pad. Keep your body off the ground with a high-quality pad underneath your sleeping bag. Even in a hammock, use a pad to protect you from the cold air circulating below you.

Get a mummy bag. I resisted buying one for years because I prefer a roomier rectangle bag. But after three freezing nights of *not* sleeping in the Andes, I finally made the switch. If you are going to be in frigid temperatures, go with this style.

Wear a single base layer. Even though it seems counterintuitive, sleeping in only one base layer is the most efficient way to stay warm. Piling on a lot of thick layers can trap humidity around your body and keep you colder. Synthetic base layers are great, but merino wool is my favorite for staying toasty!

Eat a nighttime snack. Fuel up with a slower-burning fat or protein snack just before bed. And make sure to stay hydrated.

SURVIVAL SHELTER

Knowing how to create a survival shelter is a useful skill. Follow these step-by-step instructions to build a lean-to shelter on your next campout—or even in your backyard for a spontaneous night out!

1. Look for a fallen tree or a large rock, or use your fence if you're doing a backyard adventure. A standing live tree will also work in a pinch.

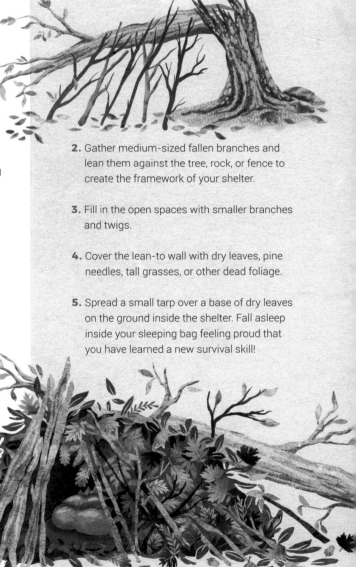

2. Gather medium-sized fallen branches and lean them against the tree, rock, or fence to create the framework of your shelter.

3. Fill in the open spaces with smaller branches and twigs.

4. Cover the lean-to wall with dry leaves, pine needles, tall grasses, or other dead foliage.

5. Spread a small tarp over a base of dry leaves on the ground inside the shelter. Fall asleep inside your sleeping bag feeling proud that you have learned a new survival skill!

WINTER CAMPING

Camping in the cold can seem intimidating. But with just a few additions to your regular gear list, you'll be able to enjoy the magical experience of waking up in your tent to a blanket of freshly fallen snow.

SLEEP SYSTEM: Invest in a high-quality down sleeping bag rated for winter. Adding a liner can increase the warmth by as much as 15 to 25 degrees. A high-R-value insulated pad will keep you from losing body heat to the cold ground. I like to toss an activated hand warmer into my bag so that it's warm when I climb in.

CLOTHING: Wear clothing made of wool or synthetic materials. Natural fabrics like cotton and denim absorb water and take a long time to dry. Pack extra base layers, a midrange puffy jacket, and a heavier winter coat so that you can adjust your layering as the temperature fluctuates.

FOOD: Your body burns more calories in colder weather so bring plenty of calorie-dense foods to stay well-fueled and warm.

GEAR: Gaiters keep snow, mud, and gravel out of your boots and protect your pant legs. Slip a set of traction cleats or microspikes onto your boots to improve your footing on snow and ice.

TIP Sleep with the next day's clothes and any batteries or electronics inside your sleeping bag. Your body heat will keep the batteries from draining, and getting dressed in the morning will be easier with warm clothes.

BUILD A QUINZEE

Similar to an igloo, this survival snow shelter originated with North American Athabaskan people. A *quinzee* is simple to construct and can be a fun place to spend the night. The interior will be just below freezing, which is quite warm if it's subzero outside! Build one for the ultimate winter camping experience:

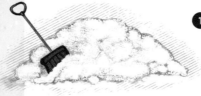

1 Shovel snow into a large mound wide enough for one or two people to sleep inside. Let the snow sit for at least two hours, giving it time to sinter (settle and solidify).

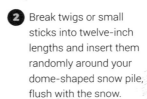

2 Break twigs or small sticks into twelve-inch lengths and insert them randomly around your dome-shaped snow pile, flush with the snow.

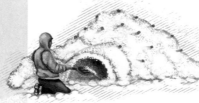

3 Begin hollowing out the entrance with a shovel. Pile the excess snow around the opening to form a windbreak.

4 Using a shovel, scoop, pot lid, or bowl, carve out the interior until you hit the ends of the guide sticks you placed around the dome. This measure ensures that your walls are at least a foot thick. Leave the sleeping area slightly raised so that cold air will sink below it.

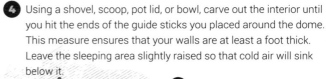

5 Poke a fist-sized ventilation hole or two through the top of the dome.

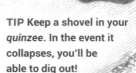

TIP Keep a shovel in your *quinzee*. In the event it collapses, you'll be able to dig out!

6 Layer the interior with a tarp, your sleeping pad, and then your sleeping bag. Enjoy a cozy night inside!

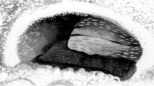

CAMPING JOURNAL

What have been some of your most memorable camping trips? Hilarious or eerie events soon become family lore, like that time you flipped the canoe and donated your phone to the lake or the night you swore you heard Bigfoot outside your tent. Write these memories down before you forget the details!

What do you love most about spending a night under the stars—watching meteors streak across the sky or waking up to fresh coffee in the forest?

Track any camping tips, tricks, and hacks you've discovered so you can use them on future trips!

TAKE THE PARK CHALLENGE

National parks are spectacular places with beautiful campgrounds, trails, wilderness, history, and diverse wildlife. There are more than sixty national parks in the US. But when you expand the definition to "national park sites," such as national monuments, national seashores, and historic sites, there are *more than four hundred!* Do you dream of visiting a specific national park— or exploring one you've been to in more depth? Recreation.gov and nps.gov are great places to begin your search. You can also go north and explore Canada's spectacular parks at www.pc.gc.ca.

What about parks closer to home? City, county, and state parks also offer a range of affordable and free amenities. When was the last time you had a cookout at a nearby city park or biked along a county greenway? Find one close to you at stateparks.org.

To take the park challenge, identify at least one park in each category and make a plan to visit it—for an overnight camping trip, a midday picnic or BBQ, or a fun family activity. Invite friends to join the challenge and discover new places together!

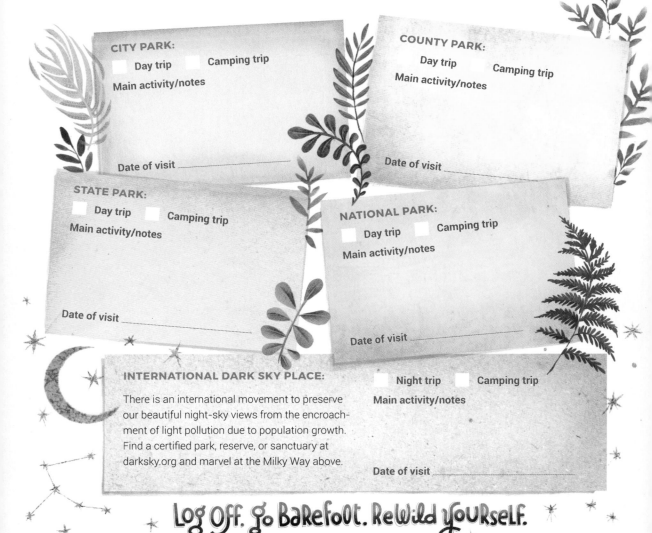

CITY PARK:
☐ Day trip   ☐ Camping trip
Main activity/notes

Date of visit _____

COUNTY PARK:
☐ Day trip   ☐ Camping trip
Main activity/notes

Date of visit _____

STATE PARK:
☐ Day trip   ☐ Camping trip
Main activity/notes

Date of visit _____

NATIONAL PARK:
☐ Day trip   ☐ Camping trip
Main activity/notes

Date of visit _____

INTERNATIONAL DARK SKY PLACE:

There is an international movement to preserve our beautiful night-sky views from the encroach-ment of light pollution due to population growth. Find a certified park, reserve, or sanctuary at darksky.org and marvel at the Milky Way above.

☐ Night trip   ☐ Camping trip
Main activity/notes

Date of visit _____

Log Off. Go Barefoot. Rewild Yourself.

MORE PARKS to EXPLORE

Keep a list of your favorite parks to check off as you visit them, or expand the park challenge to farther-flung destinations. Note special features of the park, fees, amenities, where you stayed, who came with you, and what you did in the park.

NAME / LOCATION / NOTES	TENT CAMPING	SHOWER HOUSE	RV CAMPING	PICNIC SHELTER	CABINS	TRAILS	SWIMMING	CLIMBING	SKIING	BOATING	BEACH	BIKING	HORSEBACK RIDING
1	☐	☐	☐	☐	☐	☐	☐	☐	☐	☐	☐	☐	☐
2	☐	☐	☐	☐	☐	☐	☐	☐	☐	☐	☐	☐	☐
3	☐	☐	☐	☐	☐	☐	☐	☐	☐	☐	☐	☐	☐
4	☐	☐	☐	☐	☐	☐	☐	☐	☐	☐	☐	☐	☐
5	☐	☐	☐	☐	☐	☐	☐	☐	☐	☐	☐	☐	☐
6	☐	☐	☐	☐	☐	☐	☐	☐	☐	☐	☐	☐	☐
7	☐	☐	☐	☐	☐	☐	☐	☐	☐	☐	☐	☐	☐
8	☐	☐	☐	☐	☐	☐	☐	☐	☐	☐	☐	☐	☐
9	☐	☐	☐	☐	☐	☐	☐	☐	☐	☐	☐	☐	☐
10	☐	☐	☐	☐	☐	☐	☐	☐	☐	☐	☐	☐	☐

NOTES:

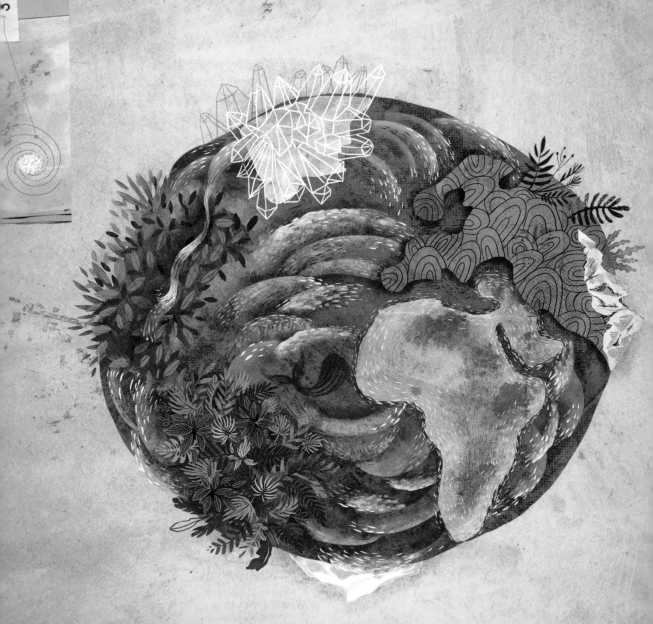

HOME.

I Haven'T been everywhere, But it's on my list.

— Susan Sontag

OUTDOOR & ADVENTURE TRAVEL

People tend to associate the phrase "outdoor adventure travel" with epic hiking, climbing, paddling, or cycling trips in far-off places. I prefer to think of it as something that pushes me out of my comfort zone, reconnects me to nature, and introduces me to people and cultures different from my own. Your travels may take you to another continent or perhaps a neighboring state. Wherever you long to go, make space in your life for travel that thrills your soul and reminds you that beauty and magic exist throughout this world.

TRAVEL AND ADVENTURE GOALS

Have you always wanted to travel to Finland to see the northern lights, stay at a Bedouin camp in the desert after a day of sandboarding, or take a cooking class in Italy or Japan? Perhaps you've dreamed of hiking in Patagonia, summiting Mount Kilimanjaro in Tanzania, or going on an underground tour in Kentucky's Mammoth Cave National Park? Make two lists below, one of *destinations* you hope to visit and another of outdoor travel *experiences* you dream about. What actions can you take to turn your lists into lifelong memories?

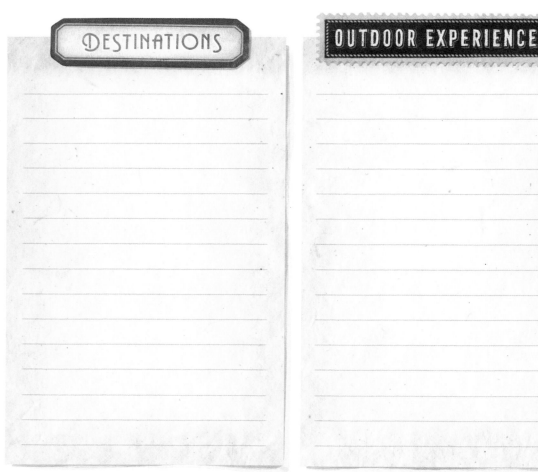

DESTINATIONS

OUTDOOR EXPERIENCES

BE SPONTANEOUS!

While you're planning, saving, and scheduling your bigger trip, have some spontaneous fun in the meantime! There are many ways to keep your outdoor adventure dreams alive, week in and week out.

DAY TRIP

Print a map of your region and make a dot where you live. Using a radius of the distance you can drive in about an hour (60 to 80 miles), draw a circle with your home at the center. Close your eyes, spin the paper, then randomly place your finger on the map: Where did it land? Go there for a day of unplanned fun!

ADVENTURE JAR

Grab a sheet of paper and jot down local adventure ideas—a hike with a view of your city, a zipline and ropes course, a bike loop with a great cafe. See if you can come up with around twenty experiences you'd love to try. Cut up the list into individual trips and put them in a jar. When you have a free day, select an idea and see where it takes you!

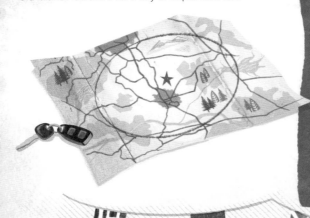

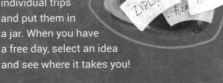

TRAVEL WEEK ... AT HOME

Can't travel? Bring the world to your home! Host an international potluck party for your book club, neighbors, family, or friends. Pick a country, region, or state and prepare dishes native to that place. For cooking inspiration and ideas, check out Global Table Adventure online.

Take your cultural immersion further by watching a movie or reading a novel set in the area. Create crafts inspired by the region's arts while listening to its native music. Download a language-learning app or consider reaching out to a local immigrant community. Is there a cultural center, restaurant, grocery store, or festival where you can meet people from a different background or part of the world? You will expand your life while celebrating global diversity!

PLAN YOUR ADVENTURE

Planning an adventure is one of my favorite parts of the journey. That said, the logistics can be overwhelming. As in the earlier "Bucket List Breakdown" exercise, it can help to break down your travel goals into approachable tasks that you can easily focus on, one step at a time. If you have a clear course of action, you can plan big adventures months or even years in advance.

Below is a basic guide (and example) to get you started. On the facing page, map out your own steps toward a specific adventure. You'll be surprised by how this simple visual exercise can help you move forward. Reevaluate as you make progress and adjust the steps as needed. Don't lose sight of your end goal: **living an adventurous life!**

PLAN YOUR GOAL:

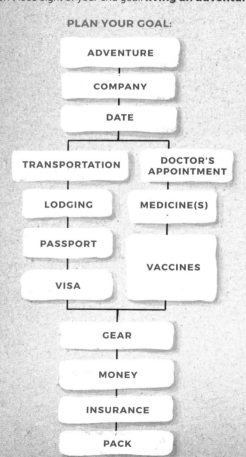

- ADVENTURE
- COMPANY
- DATE
- TRANSPORTATION — DOCTOR'S APPOINTMENT
- LODGING — MEDICINE(S)
- PASSPORT
- VISA — VACCINES
- GEAR
- MONEY
- INSURANCE
- PACK

EXAMPLE:

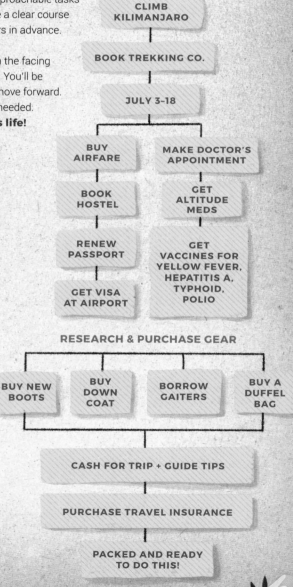

- CLIMB KILIMANJARO
- BOOK TREKKING CO.
- JULY 3–18
  - BUY AIRFARE → BOOK HOSTEL → RENEW PASSPORT → GET VISA AT AIRPORT
  - MAKE DOCTOR'S APPOINTMENT → GET ALTITUDE MEDS → GET VACCINES FOR YELLOW FEVER, HEPATITIS A, TYPHOID, POLIO

RESEARCH & PURCHASE GEAR

- BUY NEW BOOTS
- BUY DOWN COAT
- BORROW GAITERS
- BUY A DUFFEL BAG

CASH FOR TRIP + GUIDE TIPS

PURCHASE TRAVEL INSURANCE

PACKED AND READY TO DO THIS!

MAP OUT ONE ADVENTURE GOAL

Using the example at left as a model, map out your steps and set deadlines for completing each one.
Check off each finished task and celebrate your progress!

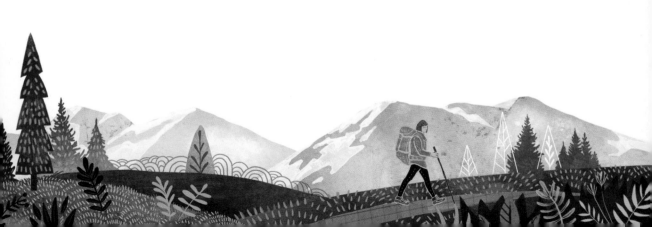

ADVENTURE BUDGET WORKSHEET

Now that you have a specific trip in mind, it's time to break down the expenses to give you an accurate idea of how much you'll need to save. Fill in an estimated cost for each item.

Calculate your monthly savings goal:
Take the total estimated cost and divide it by the number of weeks or months until your trip. For example, if you want to hike the Inca Trail and tour Cusco in eighteen months, it'll cost you about $3,000. Divided by 18, that's about $166, the amount you'll need to save each month before your trip. If that amount seems higher than your budget allows, figure out how much you can save each month and then schedule your trip based on that calculation.

Be flexible: Save for as long as you need to make your dreams happen.

Destination(s):

How many days and nights?

Airfare and transportation:

Visa or entry fees:

Immunizations:

Outfitter or tour cost
(for example, the price of a guided trek or tour):

Tips for guides, drivers, and porters:

Additional side trips and excursions beyond the main tour.

Lodging (what isn't included in the package):

Transportation
(rail pass, car or van rental, cab fares, etc.):

Food:

Travel insurance (find out if your trip requires it!):

Clothing or gear you need to purchase:

Internet access (will you use Wi-Fi, purchase a local SIM card, or use a free call app?):

Souvenirs and miscellaneous expenses:

TOTAL TRIP COST:

CHECK OUT THESE APPS AND WEBSITES TO SCORE DISCOUNTS.

Flights:
FareDrop
Skyscanner
KAYAK
momondo

Lodging:
Airbnb
Couchsurfing
Booking.com
Intervac Home Exchange

General Discounts:
Trim
Honey

Travel Deals:
Travelzoo
Groupon Experiences

Travel Expense Trackers:
Trail Wallet
Tripcoin
TrabeePocket

MONEY-SAVING TIPS AND STRATEGIES

Now that you have a monthly savings goal to work toward, consider setting up automatic monthly transfers into an account dedicated to your trip. Can you work overtime, pick up a part-time job, or take on a side hustle? Go on a spending diet and see how much you can squirrel away. Drop your gym membership and start hiking, running, or biking instead. You don't have to live an austere life to save money. Order only one drink instead of two at happy hour with friends. It takes discipline but the adventure is worth it. Here are some more suggestions to help you meet your financial goals and realize your dreams:

1. **Subscribe to travel company newsletters.** Not only will you get great location ideas, but you'll be the first to know when tours go on sale. Buy your trip during Black Friday and Cyber Monday sales when you can save hundreds of dollars. A few of my favorites are The Clymb, G Adventures, and Intrepid Travel.

2. **Look into credit card points.** "Travel hacking" is a skill, and there are plenty of websites and courses to get you started. By using certain credit cards responsibly, you can amass points that can be exchanged for free flights and hotels. WARNING: Follow this strategy only if you can pay off your balance each month so that you don't end up paying interest and fees. Check out these two sites: Kara and Nate and The Points Guy.

3. **Assess your gear needs.** Getting geared up for an adventure can be expensive, especially if you're new to an activity. Is there anything you can borrow or find used? Avoid buying new if you'll likely use a piece of gear only once.

> **BE GENEROUS.** Save money where you can, but never skimp on tips for people like guides, drivers, and porters. They are helping you create amazing memories and deserve fair compensation.

4. **Know when to buy.** Need a down coat for your big trip? Buy one at the end of winter when companies clear out their seasonal stock. The worst time for last-minute winter base layer shopping is summer, especially if you live in a warmer climate. Your local outfitter may have only a small selection in stock. Plan ahead for the best deals and options.

5. **Shop around for used gear.** Clearance is cool! Outfitters like REI frequently have garage sales where they sell used gear. Get up early and get in line. It's worth it to snag that $200 item for half price or better.

6. **Tell your family and friends about your plan.** Your family and friends are probably wondering what to get you for your birthday and the holidays. Request gift cards from gear companies, an airline, or your outfitter. They will feel happy when they see a photo of you parasailing because they helped you get there. (Except for your mom. She'll be freaking out.)

7. **Decorate a piggy bank.** Don't roll your eyes. It really works! Cover a container with photos of your dream adventure. Drop in your spare cash and watch it add up. Visualizing yourself on a beach or ski slope will make skipping your morning latte a bit easier.

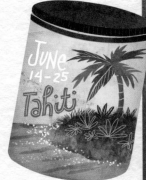

8. **Consider cheap accommodations and food.** Staying in cheaper places, such as hostels, can save you cash. You might even look into house-sitting gigs at your destination. Couch-surfing is another great option—make new friends and glean local recommendations. Instead of high-end restaurants, sample local street food for a more connected and authentic journey.

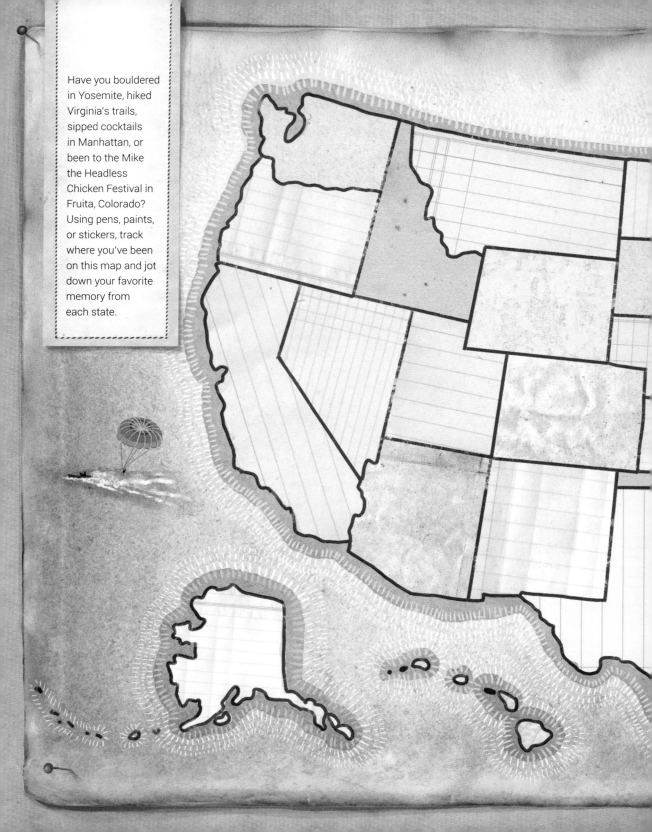

Have you bouldered in Yosemite, hiked Virginia's trails, sipped cocktails in Manhattan, or been to the Mike the Headless Chicken Festival in Fruita, Colorado? Using pens, paints, or stickers, track where you've been on this map and jot down your favorite memory from each state.

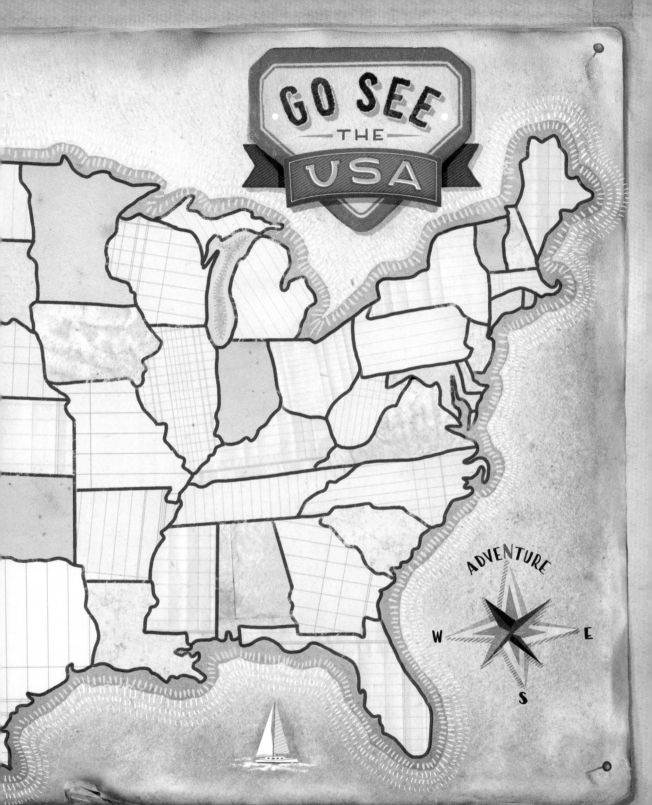

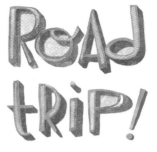

ROAD trip!

Whether you're going solo or making memories with friends, everyone should take a road trip at least once! You can eat in funky diners, marvel at weird roadside attractions, see new landscapes, and maybe even pose with a giant gas station statue of Paul Bunyan. A road trip is also a great way to discover new parks and outdoor opportunities, sometimes in unexpected places. Experience it all.

Ready to plan your next road trip? Write down some must-see destinations and fun stops along the way. Check out Roadtrippers and The Outbound Collective for adventure and lodging ideas along your route. **Be open to serendipitous detours too!**

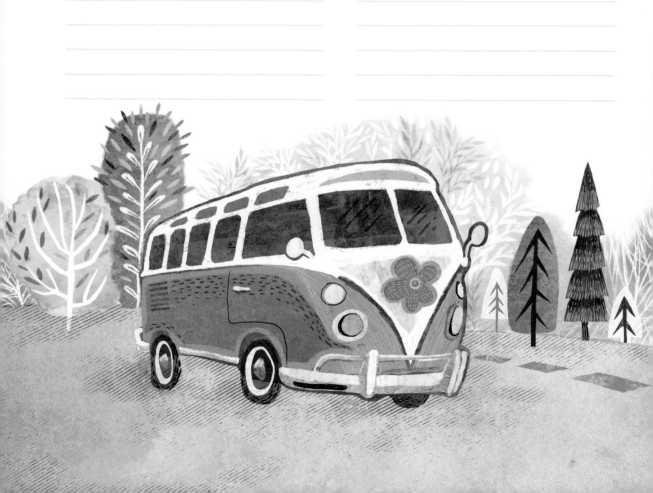

Don't forget to bring:

FAVORITE
traVeL
muG

map/GPS
APP

WateR

FLAVOR

BaKeD

Kit ROAD
SAFeTY

ComfY
Clothes

hAmmoCk

PORtable
charGer

PLaYLiSt
music, audioBooks & Podcasts

Use these pages to create a road trip log.

WHERE DID YOU GO? WHAT DID YOU DO? WHO DID YOU MEET?

THE MOST HILARIOUS THING THAT HAPPENED:

THE BEST AND WEIRDEST LOCAL FOOD I TRIED:

I'LL NEVER FORGET. . .

WELL THAT WAS UNEXPECTED. . .

WRITE ABOUT, DRAW, OR PASTE IN PHOTOS OF MORE ROAD TRIP HIGHLIGHTS:

SOLO TRAVEL

Everyone should travel alone *at least* once. Setting your own agenda and time frame allows you unparalleled freedom to redefine or even rediscover who you are. Traveling with friends or family can be rewarding, but sometimes the best way to hit the reset button is to give yourself some solo time. Focus on a personal project, take a road trip, plan an outdoor adventure, or even organize a personal retreat to recharge your soul. You'll come home refreshed, focused, and ready for more adventures!

TIPS FOR TRAVELING SOLO

I have visited five continents, mostly as a solo female traveler. The most important advice I can offer is to NOT be afraid but always be aware. All too often, women are warned not to venture out alone. And while we *do* have to take more precautions, traveling on my own has opened me up to experiences I never would have had as part of a group. I have found that locals tend to be very protective of and generous with female travelers, eager to share their culture or offer you a cup of tea.

SUGGESTIONS TO PUT YOU AT EASE:

- You have permission to start small! If you are with a group or just one other person, venture out for a solo day of exploring and see how you like it.

- When traveling abroad, register with your embassy and let them know your itinerary while in the country.

- Share your plans for the day and your expected return time with the hotel desk. Ask whether there are any areas you should avoid.

- If you are unsure about the area, arrange for a driver to pick you up from the airport and take you to your lodging.

- **TRUST YOUR GUT.** Have you ever turned a corner and gotten the feeling you shouldn't walk down that street? Listen to your instincts and find another route.

- Let friends and family back home know your plans and check in with them periodically.

SOLO TRAVEL JOURNAL

What revelations did you have about yourself? How did you feel—vibrant and alive, lonely, a bit fearful? What did you accomplish alone that you may not have with others? In what ways has your experience changed how you feel about traveling with others?

PLAN A PERSONAL RETREAT

It is essential to carve out time from our busy schedules to focus on a personal project—or ourselves. You may choose to drive to a remote cabin or simply find an Airbnb close to home.

Set your daily intention with a ritual you find meaningful. You could meditate, pray, burn incense, work with crystals, or simply sip a cup of coffee while listening to the sounds of nature. Consider undergoing a digital detox. Deleting distracting apps from your phone, even for a few days, can improve your mental energy and focus.

Before you go, mark off blocks of time in a planner for each day. Color-code your activities— move, rest, eat, sleep, fun!—and think about the timing of each: Are you mentally sharp at dawn, or do you feel most creative after midnight? Build your schedule around your natural rhythms.

Here are a few suggestions to help you organize your solo getaway.

Date and length of retreat:
Location:

What is the purpose of your retreat? What do you hope to accomplish?

Healthy foods and snacks are critical for a clear mind. What will you bring?

Move every day. Will you start your day with stretching, yoga, a hike, or a run?

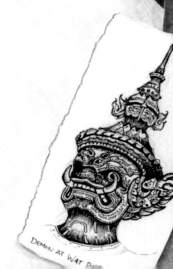

DEMON AT WAT PHO

TRAIN

No matter where you are in life, you have the power to harness one of the few things you can control in the outdoors: your fitness. Being in shape will make your adventures more enjoyable and increase your chances of success. If a summit is your goal, don't let aching quads distract you from the stunning views on the way up. And don't let fatigue decrease your margin of safety on the descent. That said, you do *not* have to be an athlete in top shape to do amazing things.

There is no need to put off your outdoor or travel goals because of your body type or current fitness level. Even if you have never set foot on a trail, consistent training will prepare you for that fall hiking getaway with friends. Start small, give yourself plenty of time, and resist frustration. Patience and persistence will get you there.

TIP Stay motivated when training by listening to audiobooks, music that energizes you, or travel podcasts from a relevant destination. While I hiked near my hometown to prepare for my trek to Everest Base Camp, adventure travel books about Nepal and Nepalese music built my anticipation and added joy to my training!

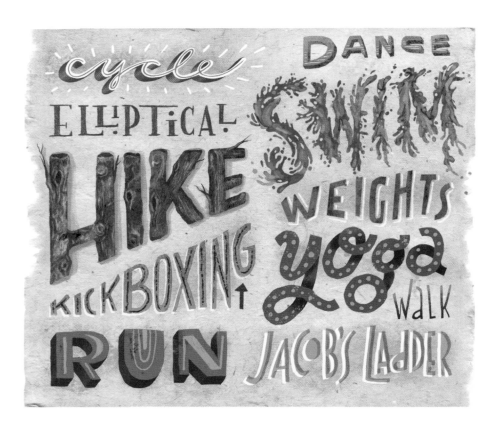

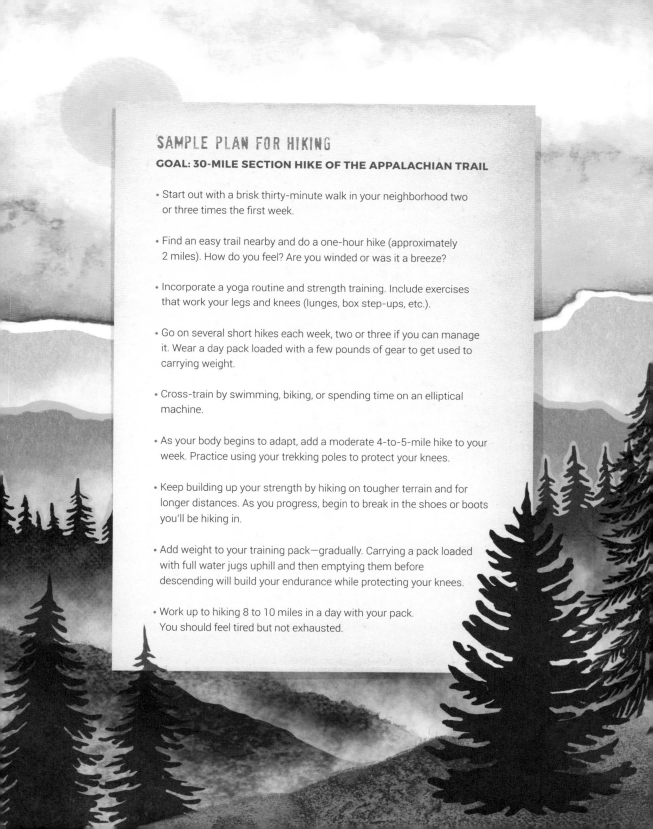

SAMPLE PLAN FOR HIKING
GOAL: 30-MILE SECTION HIKE OF THE APPALACHIAN TRAIL

- Start out with a brisk thirty-minute walk in your neighborhood two or three times the first week.

- Find an easy trail nearby and do a one-hour hike (approximately 2 miles). How do you feel? Are you winded or was it a breeze?

- Incorporate a yoga routine and strength training. Include exercises that work your legs and knees (lunges, box step-ups, etc.).

- Go on several short hikes each week, two or three if you can manage it. Wear a day pack loaded with a few pounds of gear to get used to carrying weight.

- Cross-train by swimming, biking, or spending time on an elliptical machine.

- As your body begins to adapt, add a moderate 4-to-5-mile hike to your week. Practice using your trekking poles to protect your knees.

- Keep building up your strength by hiking on tougher terrain and for longer distances. As you progress, begin to break in the shoes or boots you'll be hiking in.

- Add weight to your training pack—gradually. Carrying a pack loaded with full water jugs uphill and then emptying them before descending will build your endurance while protecting your knees.

- Work up to hiking 8 to 10 miles in a day with your pack. You should feel tired but not exhausted.

my training plan

Use this chart to craft a basic training plan for your primary outdoor sport or an upcoming race or adventure.

FITNESS GOALS:	HOW I WANT TO FEEL:	WAYS TO DRINK MORE WATER:

FIND EXERCISES YOU ENJOY AND MIX THEM UP TO CREATE YOUR ROUTINE:

SUN	MON	TUES	WED	THURS	FRI	SAT

SUN	MON	TUES	WED	THURS	FRI	SAT

GET SHAKIN'

HEALTHY FOODS I LOVE:

MY SLEEPING ROUTINE:

MY MOTIVATION:

SUN	MON	TUES	WED	THURS	FRI	SAT

DON'T STOP!

WHEN I DON'T FEEL LIKE STICKING TO THE PLAN, I WILL REPEAT THIS AFFIRMATION:

RECOVERY AND SELF-CARE

Train hard, recover harder. To absorb the benefits of your workouts, it is essential to dedicate time to recovery. Training places significant stress on your body, and too much stress without adequate rest can spell physiological disaster over time. Take a full rest day each week. Beyond that, here are a few ideas to ensure you're giving your body all the TLC it needs.

SLEEP, SLEEP, AND THEN SLEEP SOME MORE. Shoot for a full eight hours each night. Sleep is the best natural recovery tool.

EAT PLENTY AND EAT WELL. Your body needs nutritious food to repair itself after hard workouts. Try to refuel within thirty minutes to reduce next-day soreness. Your target ratio of protein to carbohydrates to fat depends on your primary activity.

STAY HYDRATED. If you struggle to drink enough water, try adding slices of fresh lemon or other fruit or all-natural flavoring mixes.

TRY YOGA. Go to a studio or flow along with an online video in the comfort of your home. All you need is a mat and an open mind to reap the benefits of this strength and mobility practice.

MEDITATE AND EXPERIMENT WITH OTHER MINDFULNESS PRACTICES. Practicing mindfulness consistently can reduce stress, increase clarity, and promote happiness. A few minutes a day can significantly affect your outlook and mental state.

SUPPLEMENT WITH OTHER MOBILITY AND MYOFASCIAL-RELEASE WORK. Use a foam roller or similar tool, get a massage from a licensed practitioner, and try other stretching exercises.

TAKE A MENTAL BREAK. Read a book, watch a TV series, take a bubble bath, or enjoy a low-key night out with friends.

TAPER! As you near your adventure goal, gradually begin to ratchet down your volume. In the final week, back way off and get ample rest, especially crucial if you are traveling abroad, because training fatigue can make you more susceptible to illness.

NIP ANY NIGGLING PAINS IN THE BUD. Take a few days off or do some cross-training instead. An overuse injury can sideline you for months. (Do the same if you feel a cold coming on.)

REMEMBER THAT STRESS IS STRESS. Your body doesn't differentiate between training stress and general life stress like work and family obligations, so cut yourself some slack when things get hectic.

The most important tip is to find an adventure that excites you. Accept where your body and fitness levels are today, then work gradually toward your goals. Healthy self-care rituals, being in nature and surrounding yourself with positive, supportive people are just the soul nourishment you need to create an amazing life.

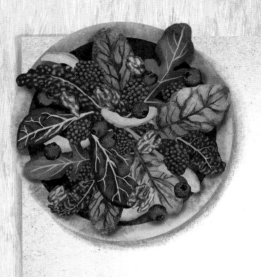

What are your favorite recovery tools? Your favorite recovery foods? What does your ideal rest day look like? Have you overcome any injuries in the past?

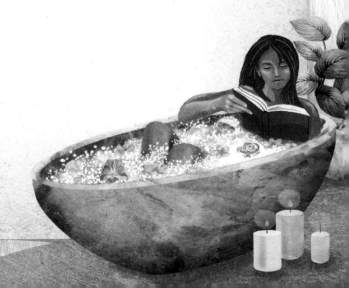

REFLECT ON YOUR OUTDOOR ADVENTURE JOURNEY

Think about these prompts as you consider your plans, fears, lists, memories, and dreams.

What have you learned about yourself?

How have your perceptions of yourself and your body changed since you started this journal?

How has your personal adventure style evolved?

What is your favorite *new* outdoor experience?

What have you done to enrich an outdoor activity you were already doing?

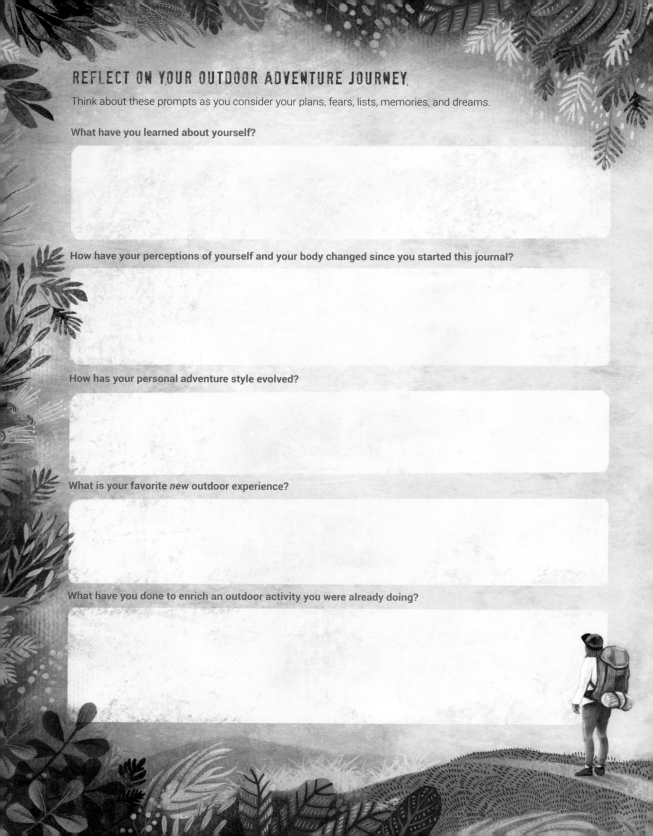

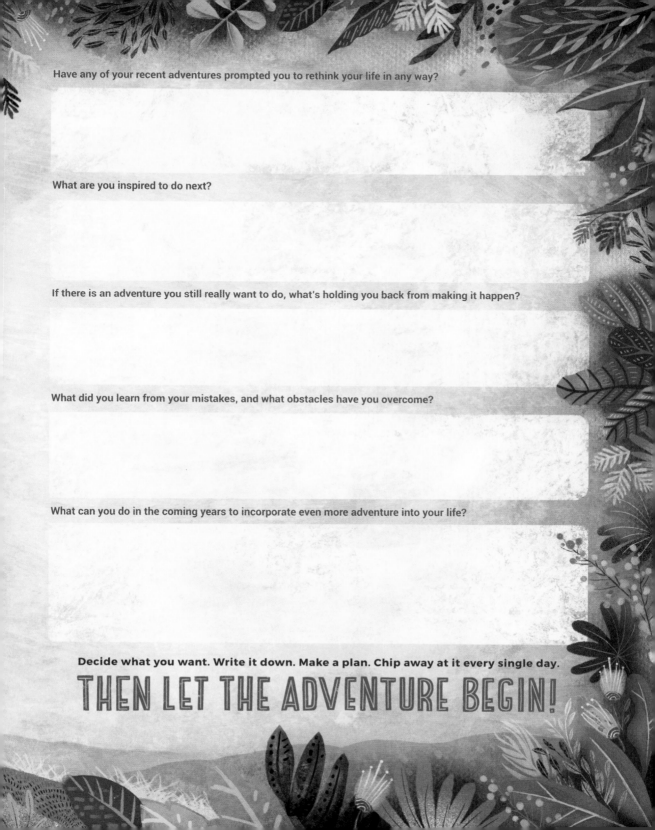

Have any of your recent adventures prompted you to rethink your life in any way?

What are you inspired to do next?

If there is an adventure you still really want to do, what's holding you back from making it happen?

What did you learn from your mistakes, and what obstacles have you overcome?

What can you do in the coming years to incorporate even more adventure into your life?

Decide what you want. Write it down. Make a plan. Chip away at it every single day.

THEN LET THE ADVENTURE BEGIN!

NOTES

Fill these pages with your plans, thoughts, custom lists, memories, and dreams.

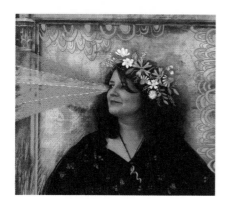

ABOUT THE AUTHOR AND ILLUSTRATOR

Illustrator and designer **SHARISSE STEBER** has collected more than thirty respected industry awards, and numerous publications have featured her art and design work. She established her career in Washington, DC, with an impressive client list that included Coca-Cola, Smithsonian Institution, The Nature Conservancy, US Postal Service, DreamWorks, NPR, the Girl Scouts, and Discovery Channel. She lives in Nashville.

www.sharissedesign.com
@sharisse_steber_design

ACKNOWLEDGMENTS

Zade. You are my favorite creation and greatest adventure. Thank you for enduring our family vacations spent sleeping on frozen lakes, camping in caves, and dangling from cliffs. Remember, I *did* take you to a beach . . . once.

My parents. Our epic family road trips showed me the world. Letting me run wild, barefoot exploring the woods alone showed me myself.

Bill and Pat. Your support for my first study abroad experience gave me the travel bug forever. Thank you.

Robert. My great love and biggest supporter—you make me feel lucky every day.

My circle of women: Lisa, Robin, Sue, Ella and Doris. Everyone should have a magical sisterhood like ours. May we always swim together in the moonlight.

My agent Jessica Alvarez. You took a chance on me and it changed everything.

My editors Kate Rogers and Laura Shauger. Your wisdom helped turn my vision into something tangible for women to live big, brave lives. I'm so grateful.

RESOURCES

Brown, Meaghen. "The Longer the Race, the Stronger We Get." *Outside* magazine online, April 11, 2017.

CNN interview with Barbara Hillary. "I Am Barbara Hillary." July 2008. www.barbarahillary.com.

Harper, Hilary. "Robyn Davidson Reflects on 40 Years Since *Tracks*." *Life Matters* podcast. Published March 30, 2018.

Hart, Scott. "Riding Up Mount Kilimanjaro: The Power of Bicycles." RedBull. Published February 6, 2018.

Khan, Gulnaz. "This Ultramarathon Runner Is Redefining What an Athlete Looks Like." *National Geographic*. March 1, 2018.

Montgomery, Ben. *Grandma Gatewood's Walk: The Inspiring Story of the Woman Who Saved the Appalachian Trail.* Chicago: Chicago Review Press, 2014.

Pharr Davis, Jennifer. "Positive Forward Motion." YouTube. Published May 6, 2020.

Yoshikawa, Mai. "Mountain Queen Not Done Yet." *The Japan Times*. February 25, 2003.

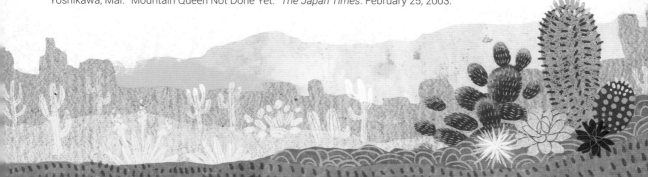

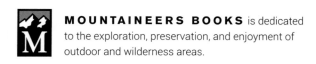

MOUNTAINEERS BOOKS is dedicated to the exploration, preservation, and enjoyment of outdoor and wilderness areas.

1001 SW Klickitat Way, Suite 201, Seattle, WA 98134
800-553-4453, www.mountaineersbooks.org

Printed in China
Distributed in the United Kingdom by Cordee, www.cordee.co.uk
24 23 22 21   1 2 3 4 5

Copyeditor: Laura Case Larson
Design and layout: Sharisse Steber
Production Artist: Robert Bright

Mountaineers Books titles may be purchased for corporate, educational, or other promotional sales, and our authors are available for a wide range of events. For information on special discounts or booking an author, contact our customer service at 800-553-4453 or mbooks@mountaineersbooks.org.

Printed on FSC®-certified materials

FSC
www.fsc.org
MIX
Paper from responsible sources
FSC® C008047

ISBN: 978-1-68051-522-0

An independent nonprofit publisher since 1960

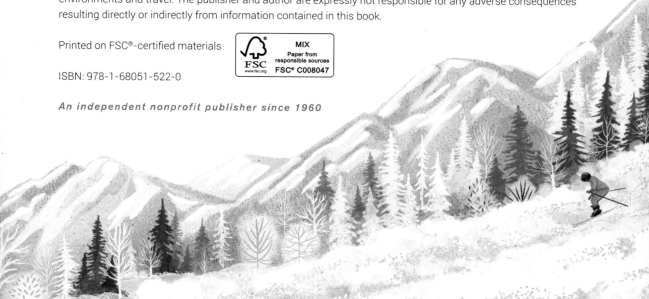